ercise your way to health:
ıck pain

cise plans to improve your life

dedication

For Mum and Dad

exercise your way to health:
back pain

exercise plans to improve your life

Paula Coates

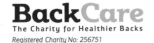

Note
Whilst every effort has been made to ensure that the content of this book is as technically accurate and as sound as possible, neither the author nor the publishers can accept responsibility for any injury or loss sustained as a result of the use of this material.

Published in 2010 by
A & C Black Publishers Ltd
36 Soho Square, London W1D 3QY
www.acblack.com

Copyright © 2010 Paula Coates

ISBN 978 14081 0703 4

A CIP catalogue record for this book is available from the British Library.

Acknowledgements
Cover photograph © Shutterstock
Inside photographs © Grant Pritchard, except p 4 iStockphotos.com,
  pp 24, 34, 36, 60, 82 Shutterstock
Illustrations by Jeff Edwards, except p 44 Mark Silver
Designed by James Watson
Commissioned by Charlotte Croft
Edited by Kate Turvey

This book is produced using paper that is made from wood grown in managed, sustainable forests. It is natural, renewable and recyclable. The logging and manufacturing processes conform to the environmental regulations of the country of origin.

Typeset in 9.25pt AGaramond on 12pt by Margaret Brain.

Printed and bound in China by WKT

contents

acknowledgements   vi
foreword   vii
endorsement   viii
introduction   1
    what can I do if I have back pain?   2

part 1: everything you need to know about your spine   5
what is back pain?   5
signs and symptoms   6
your spine and how it works   7
what causes my back pain?   15
what puts me at risk?   20
screening and diagnosis   21

part 2: helping yourself to health   25
where do I start?   25
your personal MOT   26
healthy eating   33
stopping smoking   36
good posture   39
pacing yourself   46
what help can I get?   50

part 3: the exercises   61
where do I start?   61
before you start   63
getting back to fitness: home routine   69
getting back to fitness: swimming   77
getting back to fitness: taking it outdoors   80
exercises for your back   86

find out more   117

acknowledgements

I would like to say a big thank you to all those who have given their time and support to me during the writing of this book – family, friends, and colleagues alike. A special thank you to all my patients who have been my greatest teachers and have allowed their experiences to be included in this book. Finally, a big thank you to Charlotte Croft and Kate Turvey at A&C Black, my models and Grant Pritchard for his photography.

foreword

I am delighted to be able to write a foreword to this timely and extremely useful book. We live in an ever more complex world and our lives are surrounded by gadgets and devices, all of which come with commensurately large instruction manuals, although I suspect most of us only ever look at a small handful of the instructions enclosed therein.

Against this background we all live our lives with an anatomical structure which is far more complex in structure and function than all of these seemingly complicated gadgets: our spine. It protects our spinal cord, carries a large amount of weight for 70 years or more, somehow maintains an extremely wide range of movement, contributes substantially to our shape and creates our physical identity in the eyes of others. It is amazing, therefore, that so few of us have any real insight into what should be called a 'user's manual' for the spine and that is why this book is timely and very helpful. Paula Coates is a well-respected and experienced musculoskeletal physiotherapist and her overall view of anatomy, function, how to look after our spines when they are healthy, and how to self-manage in an holistic fashion when they are hurting, will serve brilliantly as the 'user's manual' for the vertebral column.

Her philosophy of general fitness, posture, awareness of the significance of symptoms, and simple treatment and management strategies will help anybody suffering with a back problem and should probably be compulsory reading for everybody, even in the absence of symptoms. I hope you enjoy reading this book and will come back to it whenever your spine causes you concern over the years.

John O'Dowd FRCS Orth
Consultant Orthopaedic Surgeon
Director, Real Health Institute

endorsement

As a busy working GP and musculoskeletal specialist I can highly recommend this book as essential reading for patients and clinicians alike. This book is well researched, concise and up-to-date, and written by a first rate, highly experienced physiotherapist. It will give much needed and added support for patients with back pain who want to do all they can to understand and manage their condition.

Dr Gregor McEwan MB BS Dip Sports Med Lon

introduction

The management of acute and chronic back pain has been a big part of my working life for many years. It is one of the most common pains that most of us experience at some point in our lives, so it is important to understand the causes and how you can manage it. I hope this book will be a starting point to help you understand your pain and how you can deal with it day-to-day.

The idea for this book first came to me when I had severe back and leg pain a few years ago. As a physiotherapist specialising in back pain, I knew what I was supposed to do to help myself. But practising what I preach was far from easy – even though I had instant access to treatment and medication from my colleagues, and the reassurance from the information I give my patients every day. Through my exercise programme and managing my health I regained my fitness and completed four marathons. You may not be as keen on running as me, but managing your health and improving your fitness can have a significant impact on your back pain and help you to achieve your goals. This book is designed to provide you with reassurance and information as you help yourself through the bad bits, and advice on when and where to seek help if you need it. The book aims to:

- teach you the facts about back pain

- dispel the myths about back pain

- show you how to manage your back pain in the acute and non-acute phases

- give you a spinal stability exercise programme to build into your lifestyle

- alert you to the warning signs of a serious problem

- help you understand and avoid the stress and anxiety associated with back pain

- allow you to get on with your everyday life.

The book is split into three main parts. **Part 1** covers everything that you need to know about your spine, including the answers to questions I have been asked many times by my patients over the years. Once you know exactly what you are dealing with, it is much easier to formulate a plan to manage your back pain.

Part 2 looks at what you can do to help yourself: the changes you can make to your lifestyle that will help you become fitter, healthier and in control of your own health. It also explains where to ask for advice and what help is available if you need it.

Part 3 covers the exercises you can use to strengthen your body and help prevent future problems. Prevention is always better than cure, and usually much less painful. I will show you the exercises that will help you manage your pain and return to fitness, no matter how unfit you may be. I will also show you how to monitor your own progress with simple tests that you can perform at home. When you see the results of adding exercise to your life you will wish you had done so sooner.

what can I do if I have back pain?

Millions of people live with acute and chronic back pain. Although most lead a full and active life by adapting their lifestyles in response to their symptoms, many people with back pain don't achieve this – they give up work and are unable to do the things they want to. However, this does not have to be the case. By increasing your understanding of your condition and how you can help yourself to health, you can improve the quality of your life.

Chronic back pain can affect your health over a long time. When you are first diagnosed it is easy to feel overwhelmed and as if the condition will take over your life, especially if you need to take daily medication. It's important to understand that you have a choice about your condition becoming a serious problem. You can take steps to

'I was convinced there was something really wrong with my back when the pain was so severe. But as things settled and I understood more about what can cause pain, I discovered how important knowing the facts about back pain was and how much I can do myself to make things better.'

Katherine, London

control the negative effects of back pain on your health. Believe this, and by engaging in active self-management you will see the benefits of making changes to your lifestyle. When you take care of your body, it will take care of you and prevent problems in the future.

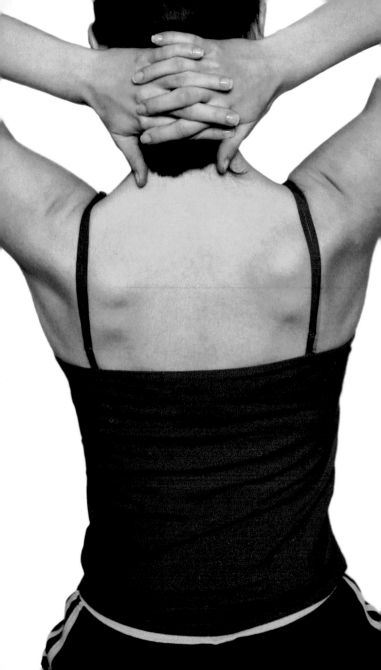

part 1
everything you need to know about your spine

what is back pain?

Back pain is one of the most common types of pain – 80 per cent of us will experience it at some point in our lifetime. It is probably as common and naturally occurring in humans as grey hair and wrinkles. You are most likely to suffer from a significant episode of back pain between the ages of 30 and 50, but mechanical back pain is also seen in children and teenagers. To put it into perspective, if you have back pain you are not alone. However severe your pain, you are experiencing something that happens to most people at some point in their life.

It is very unlikely that any two people will present with identical back pain symptoms, and usually everyone will require a different management programme, tailored to his or her individual circumstances. Please don't be panicked by stories you hear from people who paint a bleak picture of back pain. For every story of doom and gloom you hear, I can tell you another of someone who has experienced terrible pain and worked hard to get back to fitness, restore their spinal stability and live a full working and sporting life.

signs and symptoms

common symptoms

Pain: Pain is an experience personal to each individual. *The Textbook of Pain* (ed. P. D. Wall and R. Melzack, Churchill Livingstone, Edinburgh, 1999) describes pain as 'an unpleasant sensory and emotional experience associated with actual or potential tissue damage, or described in terms of such damage'. I have learnt to accept my patients' own descriptions of their pain – so if someone says it's like spiders or knives in their back, so be it! Diagnosing the cause of your back pain is based on characterising pain in various ways, according to its duration, intensity, type (dull, burning or stabbing) and location in your body.

Restricted movement: Being unable to move, or do basic things like getting dressed, is a common symptom of back pain. Muscle spasm – which is basically your muscle overworking – is a major cause of movement restriction because your muscles tighten and become overprotective when you experience pain. This can be painful in itself, and it is also important to recognise when fear of moving is part of the problem, since fear will hold you back from recovery as much as anything else.

Altered sensation: This is common and can vary from numbness or pins and needles in your arms or legs, to one limb feeling odd or just different from the other one. Some people describe an oversensitivity in the leg (or arm, if the neck is the problem area) rather than numbness. These are all symptoms that should be checked before you are treated.

Weakness: Weakness in your legs can be caused by inflammation or compression of a nerve in your back. It can also be caused by pain, which can prevent you from using your muscles normally. Physiotherapists, osteopaths and chiropractors (see page 50) will all test both your muscle strength and nerve function before you receive any treatment for back and leg pain, to see whether a nerve is being compressed and to make sure you get the right treatment.

more serious symptoms

Bladder and bowel problems: Incontinence and/or urine retention are two symptoms that must not be ignored, no matter how embarrassing telling someone may seem. If these symptoms have come on with your back pain, seek medical advice immediately.

Unexplained weight loss: Weight loss can occur for many reasons, but if it is unexplained and you haven't been on a diet, it could be a sign that something is wrong. Your GP is the best person to see and will be able to assess you further to find out why you are losing weight.

Night pain: Most pain will settle when you are lying down and you will experience some relief, even if it is only for short periods. However, if your pain becomes more severe when you are in bed at night or lying down, you should see your doctor.

Sweats: Hot sweats during the day or at night can have many causes, but if they are new to you and have come on as you have developed back pain it is important to see your doctor.

your spine and how it works

The spine is made up of 33 vertebrae. Each vertebra is attached to the one above and below it by ligaments and muscles, and is separated from the vertebrae above and below it by an intervertebral disc (fig. 1.1).

Figure 1.2 shows how the vertebrae sit together to form the whole spine. The pelvis attaches to the bottom of the spine and together they create the strong structure from which your arms and legs are hung. All the bones of the spine are held together by strong ligaments, and these are supported by the deep muscles that form part of the core muscles which give your spine stability and strength.

ligaments

The ligaments, which sit deep and close to the spine, have their own nerve supply and can be responsible for back pain if strained or sprained, very similar to the pain if you sprain your ankle. As the intervertebral discs age they become narrow, and this can affect how

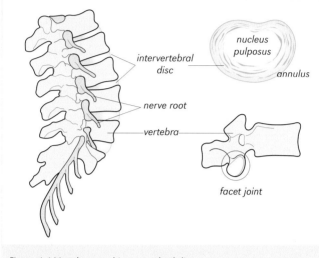

Figure 1.1 Vertebrae and intervertebral discs

well the ligaments work. If they can't control the movement between the bones in the spine, the strength of your deep spinal muscles becomes more important. This is why maintaining spinal stability and muscle control as we age is helpful in managing pain.

discs

Discs act like shock absorbers to cushion the compression between your vertebrae and also to limit the rotation and bending needed in everyday movement of your spine. They get much of the blame for back pain since it was discovered that they can prolapse or herniate – medical terms, both meaning the same thing, for a 'slipped disc'. This means that the soft nucleus of the disc has leaked through a tear in the stronger outer layer (the annulus). This is not always caused by a sudden movement, but can be the result of the normal process of disc dehydration as you age. It is not necessarily painful: many people have a disc prolapse and don't ever know it. However, if your disc herniates and the nucleus seeps through the annulus, the nucleus will take up

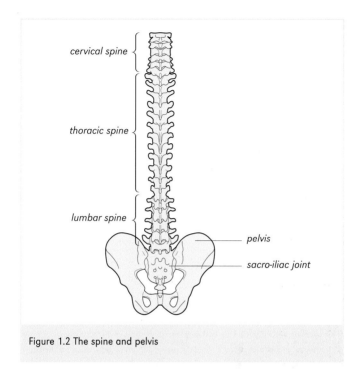

Figure 1.2 The spine and pelvis

space in your spinal canal or the space where your spinal nerves sit. If this happens, you may have pain in your back and legs.

myths about discs

The term 'slipped disc' is a misnomer, as discs themselves don't slip. However, once the central part of a disc (the nucleus) leaks through the outer layer (annulus), it can't go back in. Similarly, discs don't crumble, but small tears occur around the annulus as part of the normal ageing process. Annular tears are also a common cause of back pain (fig. 1.3).

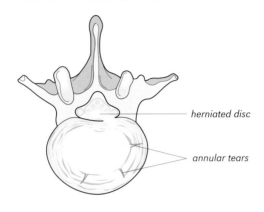

Figure 1.3 Herniated disc and annular tears

spinal canal

The spinal canal contains the spinal cord. Your spinal cord is covered by a membrane called a dural sheath which also contains the fluid that nourishes the cord and the brain. The cord comprises all the nerves that send signals from the brain to the rest of the body and back again. This includes the nerves that send pain signals to the brain and send signals to contract or relax your muscles. The spinal nerves come off the spinal cord in pairs at each vertebral level and sit in their own channel. As we age, the spinal canal can become narrowed by arthritis and this can cause pain as it reduces the space available for the spinal cord. This is called spinal stenosis.

facet joints

The facet joints are formed between the upper and lower bony projections on the lamina (bony wings) of each vertebra (see fig. 1.4).

These joints limit backwards bending and twisting, to protect the disc from too much strain. A thin layer of cartilage, a type of connective tissue, sits on the surface of your joints. This acts as a cushion and also

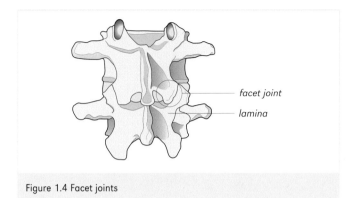

facet joint

lamina

Figure 1.4 Facet joints

allows smooth movement. Inside your joint capsule there is a small amount of synovial fluid, which acts like engine oil to help the joint move smoothly.

Arthritis, which occurs with the normal wear of the joint surface, is common in facet joints. It can cause a gradual thickening of the joint as more bone is laid down in response to overloading and pressure.

muscles

The many muscles associated with your spine (see fig. 1.5) all have a specific role to play in creating stability and movement. The deeper muscles, commonly referred to as the 'core stability' muscles or 'muscular corset', stabilise your spine. When you have back pain these muscles often stop working properly, making your spine feel weaker and less well supported.

The bigger and stronger muscles in your body lie over the top of the core stability muscles and are closer to the surface. They have the role of moving your body, while the deeper muscles support the spine. When you have back pain, some of these movement muscles can go into spasm and restrict your movement. Muscle spasm alone can be very painful and if left untreated will feed into a vicious cycle of pain and loss of movement.

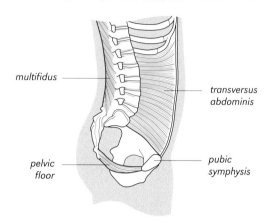

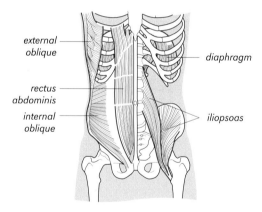

Figure 1.5 The main muscles associated with the spine: the core stability muscles (above) and key movement muscles (below)

What is muscle spasm?

Muscle spasm is an involuntary contraction of a muscle that usually results in pain and stiffness and can be caused by:

- dehydration
- muscle strain
- pain and inflammation
- trauma or injury
- poor posture.

It responds well to heat, massage and acupuncture, but you can prevent spasm in your back by having good posture and keeping yourself well hydrated.

Deep core stability muscles:

- are continuously 'switched on' – working to stabilise your spine

- are close to the joints in your spine

- stabilise your spine as you move.

These muscles form the muscular corset that helps support your spine and makes it strong. The key muscles working to support your back are:

- the transverse abdominis, the deepest of the abdominal muscles, which acts rather like the buckle on a belt
- the multifidus, which forms the back part of the muscular corset

- the pelvic floor, which acts like a sling at the bottom of the pelvis

- the diaphragm, which helps you breathe in and out.

Research has shown that having strong core muscles reduces lower back pain. They need to work together to keep your trunk stable and improve your balance, enabling you to put more effort into arm and leg movements. If the core muscles are weak, other muscles have to work harder to compensate and this can lead to muscle imbalances.

Movement muscles:

- are not close to the joints of the spine

- allow your body to move but can also go into spasm

- work with the core stability muscles to strengthen, move and stabilise your spine. I will show you how to exercise to strengthen these muscles in part 3.

Key muscles are:

- the rectus abdominis – better known as the 'six pack' – a long flat muscle, which sits along the length of the front of your tummy

- the external obliques, which flex and rotate the spine, and lie on top of the internal obliques and above the transverse abdominal muscle

- the internal obliques, which act as an opposing muscle (an 'antagonist') to the diaphragm

- the iliopsoas, a strong muscle which attaches to the front of the vertebrae and on to the thigh bone. It pulls on your thigh bone helping to bring your knee to your chest or your chest to your knees.

Other muscles that help with spinal stability and strengthening your spine are the muscles in your back, buttocks and around your pelvis and hips. These are sometimes referred to as the 'outer core' or the front and back 'slings' and they assist stabilisation and help your body move. There is a great stretch called the 'crucifix' (page 106) which helps keep these muscles flexible and supporting your back.

what causes my back pain?

The causes of back pain fall under three umbrellas. Within each there are different conditions. I will talk about these and what you can do to manage each later in the book. The three types of back pain are:

- **mechanical problems** such as muscular strains and sprains

- **nerve irritation** from the disc, ligament or facet joint

- **serious spinal pathology** such as infection or tumour.

Before you decide you have a serious spinal pathology, here are a few figures that will reassure you. Your pain may be severe, but the level of pain does not always equate with something serious. The figures for the number of people diagnosed under each of the umbrellas are:

- 93 per cent mechanical low back pain

- 5 per cent nerve root pathology

- 2 per cent serious spinal pathology.

Pain caused by the spine is not always felt in the back: many people suffer with associated leg pain, or referred pain, which is also called sciatica. This can sometimes be worse than the pain in your back, and it is important to know what is causing it to ensure it is treated effectively. Causes of leg pain can be:

- nerve root irritation or compression of a nerve in your back

- nerve irritation or compression away from your spine (in your buttock or leg)

- an injury to your leg unrelated to your back pain.

common causes

There are many reasons why you may have back pain. Some are obvious, some creep up on you over time, and some are very easy to prevent. The most common causes of back pain I have treated over the years are:

- **poor posture**

- **poor lifting technique**

- **poor ergonomics** – how your workstation is set up, whether in the workplace or at home

- **stress** – this affects everyone differently and it is important to be aware how stress manifests itself in you

- **poor mattress** – how old is your mattress, and is it supporting you?

- **deconditioning** – after illness, injury or using crutches you won't be as strong or as fit as before, and back pain can be a side-effect

- **a busy life**

- **pregnancy** – this can have a huge effect on your posture as you're carrying such a heavy weight in front of you

- **arthritis** – this is not always painful, but if you have some arthritis in your spine it can flare up from time to time

- **trauma** – anything from a fall on a slippery pavement to a car accident can result in acute or chronic pain.

less common causes
disc herniation

This occurs when a disc between the vertebrae bulges and can push against nerves and ligaments in the spine. There are three types of disc herniation/prolapse (fig 1.6), all of which produce different symptoms.

The normal ageing of a disc will lead to dehydration and a reduction in its height. The nucleus should sit centrally in the disc and most people's nucleus will stay central as they age. The different stresses and strains that your spine goes through in a lifetime will influence how the position of the nucleus may change and how it may bulge or become herniated.

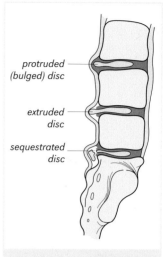

protruded (bulged) disc

extruded disc

sequestrated disc

Figure 1.6 Types of herniated disc

- **A protruded/bulging disc**, the most common type of disc herniation, is when the soft inner centre of the disc moves towards the edge of the disc and pushes against the outer shell. The bulging disc can push against ligaments and nerves, and cause inflammation which leads to back pain. Many factors can contribute to causing a disc to bulge including lifestyle, posture, poor lifting technique and lack of general fitness. It is rarely the result of just one thing or event. Manual therapy, acupuncture, physiotherapy rehabilitation and exercise will help manage this kind of pain.

- **An extruded disc** is the next stage, in which the nucleus bulges through a tear in the disc wall and pushes on the adjacent spinal nerve roots and ligaments. This process can create a lot of inflammation and subsequent pain. Extruded discs create a greater risk of nerve root irritation and compression which can cause leg pain (sciatica). Manual therapy, acupuncture, physiotherapy and specific exercises will help manage this kind of pain. If the symptoms indicate serious compression on the nerve root, further treatment may be needed and it may take longer to recover. In most cases surgery will not be required.

- **A sequestrated disc** occurs when the extruded part of the disc breaks off. This can give many symptoms which can be severe and changeable as the piece of floating disc moves. This sometimes, though not always, requires surgery.

spinal stenosis

This is caused when the spinal canal narrows, usually as a result of arthritis. The condition develops over many years and can cause pain as it reduces the space available for the spinal cord. If your doctor or physiotherapist suspects you may have spinal stenosis, X-rays and an MRI scan will confirm the diagnosis and allow it to be monitored and managed effectively.

spondylolisthesis

This is a rare problem and affects under 5 per cent of people with back pain. It is diagnosed by an X-ray showing that a lumbar vertebra has moved forwards or backwards slightly from its normal alignment.

There are two kinds of spondylolisthesis. The most common occurs over the age of 50 and is a result of the postural stresses your spine has had in life. It is seen more in women and people of African origin than in Caucasians. It progresses slowly over many years. This kind of spondylolisthesis is unlikely to need surgery unless the nerves become irritated by the spinal canal becoming narrowed. Natural fusion (the discs becoming fixed and ridged) commonly occurs and movement between the two vertebrae is reduced as a result.

The second kind of spondylolisthesis, known as spondylolysis, occurs in children due to a bone defect in the vertebra. It is caused by a crack in the bone or a failure of the bone to form and if it occurs on both sides of the vertebra the bony process can no longer restrain the weight of the body and the vertebra moves forward. This problem needs close monitoring and occasionally requires surgery, in which screws are used to fix the vertebrae in place and prevent them from moving any further forward.

cauda equina syndrome

The cauda equina is the collective name given to the spinal nerves as they come out of the bottom of the spinal cord. If the nerves are compressed at this level by a disc herniating backwards towards your spinal cord, cauda equina syndrome is possible. It is more common for the disc to herniate to one side or the other rather than backwards or forwards, but all directions are possible. If the cauda equina does become compressed, you may not be able to empty your bladder or may lose control of your bowels. You may also experience numbness in your genital area.

Cauda equina syndrome is uncommon, but if you have these symptoms they need immediate medical attention. This is the only time you should go to A&E with back pain. The earlier you are assessed and treated, the better chance your nerve has of recovering.

osteoporosis

Osteoporosis is caused by a progressive loss of strength in the bone due it losing its mineral density. This makes the bone brittle and more prone to fracture, even from minor bumps and falls. It can be managed with medication and lifestyle changes, but it is important to be diagnosed so you can minimise the risk of fractures.

Osteoporosis is most common in women after the menopause due to the reduction in the amount of oestrogen produced by the body. However, men can also suffer from it, and it can also occur in people with hormonal disorders or chronic disease, or who are taking certain medication such as steroids.

Vertebral fractures due to osteoporosis will cause sudden severe pain, often with shooting pain caused by nerve compression. This can lead to a stooped posture and reduced mobility.

Daily supplements of calcium and vitamin D are recommended, together with regular weight-bearing exercise. Medical treatments focus on stopping or slowing down mineral loss, and include:

- oral biphosphonates (such as Fosamax and Actonel), usually the first line of treatment for women

- Raloxifene (Evista), an oestrogen receptor which attracts oestrogen in the body to help prevent bone loss and fracture – helpful if you cannot tolerate bisphosphonates

- synthetic parathyroid hormone (Forsteo), used for men or postmenopausal women with severe hip or spinal osteoporosis.

Hormone replacement therapy, once widely used, is no longer used to prevent osteoporosis after the menopause, but is recommended for young women who no longer have periods.

back pain in children
Back pain in children is usually mild and a result of poor posture or growth spurts (growing pains) which are caused when bone and muscle development are not happening at the same rate. In very sporty children who repetitively put their spine through stress and strain, for example fast bowling in cricket, there may be a risk of stress fracture to the bony arch called the *pars interarticularis*, which is a part of the vertebrae. This will be diagnosed by an MRI scan. Rest with physiotherapy and rehabilitation over three to six months may be needed, but surgery is rarely required.

scoliosis and curvatures
Scoliosis is a side-to-side curve in the spine rather than the normal front to back curve. This may or may not cause any more trouble than normal spinal anatomy.

If you think you or your child has a scoliosis it's a good idea to have it checked out. It doesn't mean you or they will have any more episodes of back pain than anyone else, but you still need to watch your posture both standing and sitting and keep fit to ensure good spinal health.

what puts me at risk?
Some of the predisposing factors to getting back pain are:

- **Being female:** Women are slightly more vulnerable to back pain, although why this should be so is unclear. One suggestion is that back pain can be influenced by changes in hormones, for example during and after pregnancy and childbirth. Lifting, carrying and breastfeeding children are also major contributing factors.

- **Poor diet:** Eating a diet which is high in fat can lead to fatty deposits in the arteries (atherosclerosis), which affects circulation. Research has shown that people with atherosclerosis are more likely to have disc degeneration, leading to a higher risk of developing back pain.

- **Smoking:** It is well documented that smoking has a negative effect on health and leads to poor circulation and atherosclerosis. Along with the increased risk of back pain, smokers heal much more slowly, which will affect you if you have inflammation, an injury or surgery.

- **Poor posture.**

It is a common misconception that being overweight makes you more at risk of developing your first episode of back pain. In fact, tall people are more likely to develop back pain due to the length of the spine, which increases the pull and leverage on their lumbar spine.

Surprisingly, you are just as likely to develop back pain if you are fit – which can be a real shock if you are a fit person. The good news is that muscle strength and general fitness do prevent the recurrence of low back pain and reduce the impact of chronic back pain on day-to-day life.

screening and diagnosis

If you have seen your doctor a few times about your back pain, or it is failing to improve with treatment, he or she may request tests to find out more about what is causing your pain. For most people who have back pain these investigations are not necessary. Some of the tests that are commonly requested to investigate back pain are:

X-rays

X-ray images reveal the bony architecture of your spine and are useful for showing:

- narrowing of the disc space, which means the disc is dehydrated

- arthritis in the facet joints

- osteoporosis (thinning and reduced bone density)

- bone spurs around the vertebrae.

It is not advisable to have too many X-rays, because of the doses of radiation required to create images of the spine.

magnetic resonance imaging (MRI)

MRI uses magnetic and radio waves to create an image of the body. You lie inside a large, cylinder-shaped magnet, which passes powerful magnetic waves through the body. MRI scans are used to look at:

- bone and disc structure

- the disc position in relation to the spinal cord and nerves

- muscle tissue and fatty deposits within muscles

- the size and shape of the spinal canal.

bone scan

In some cases, your doctor may refer you to a specialist for a bone scan. A bone scan is very useful when it is unclear exactly where the problem lies, as it reveals trouble spots on the spine. A radioactive chemical, sometimes called a 'tracer', is injected into the bloodstream. The chemical attaches itself to areas of the skeleton that are making new bone, and a special camera takes pictures of these. Concentrations of the tracer, which appear as dark spots, usually indicate a problem. Your doctor may then order additional tests to find out more. A bone scan can show problems such as:

- bone tumours

- infection

- fractures

- bone density and the bone thinning seen in osteoporosis.

The test for osteoporosis uses a different type of scan which doesn't require the injection of a tracer.

computerized tomography (CT) scanning

CT scanning can give clear pictures not only of bones but of soft tissues such as muscles, organs, large blood vessels and nerves, none of which show up on an X-ray. CT scans are used:

- to detect tumours, abscesses or abnormal blood vessels, when they are suspected by symptoms or other tests

- to give a surgeon a clear picture of an area of your body before certain types of surgery

- to pinpoint the exact site of tumours before radiotherapy.

blood tests

Blood tests may help rule out other causes of back pain, such as inflammatory arthritis or infection. They will also pick up any other serious condition that may be an underlying cause of your back pain.

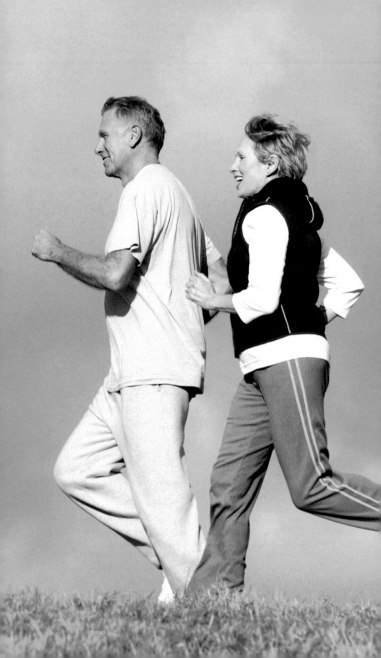

part 2

helping yourself to health

where do I start?

The first thing to think about is what you can do to help yourself. To help you do this, this part of the book begins with an MOT quest-ionnaire on page 27. The aim is to focus on your fitness and what you are currently doing to manage your pain. This is followed by advice on various self-help strategies: how to eat healthily; stop smoking; improve your posture when you are standing, lifting, sitting and sleeping; pace yourself and embrace the concept of 'active rest'; and self-medicate where possible. Finally there is advice on where to seek help if you need it, and what prescription medications or other treatments are available.

As you read through this section you will see I have used a traffic light system of treatment options. This is designed to make it easy for you to understand the options available for back pain and which is most appropriate for you.

> 'I am so much better than I was and that is all down to exercise, improving my core stability and trusting my physiotherapist, even on the days when I didn't want to believe she had no cure. I still get bad days but that doesn't mean a day off work – I just pace myself and keep moving.'
>
> Richard, London

The traffic lights work as follows:

Green

Go ahead: this is the self treatment you can start immediately to manage your injury and prevent it from becoming worse.

Amber

Proceed with caution: you may need assessment and treatments that a physiotherapist or health care professional may advise to manage your flare-up.

Red

Stop! Things are serious and need assessment to rule out complications and you may need to take advice on the best way to manage things this time.

The last thing that may come to mind when you are in pain is exercise, but there are many different ways to exercise and different levels of fitness that can be achieved as your pain settles down. Part 3 shows you exactly what exercises will help you manage your back pain and improve your fitness.

your personal MOT

Even if you have had back pain for many years, it's worth checking your current level of health and fitness. If you have been newly diagnosed with mechanical back pain, then you definitely need to give some thought to your exercise history so that you can start or continue to exercise and avoid aggravating your symptoms.

The questions below are designed to give you a brief MOT. The questionnaire is not designed to give you a full medical check-up – only a professional can do that, so visit your GP or a physiotherapist if you are significantly overweight, unable to control your back pain or have other ongoing medical problems. Your MOT will help you to focus on your general health and your back pain, spotting the tell-tale signs of potential problems that may be lurking just around the corner. Answer the questions as honestly as you can.

MOT questionnaire

	yes	no
1 Would you describe yourself as unfit?		
2 Would you describe yourself as overweight?		
3 Are you off work because of your back pain?		
4 Are you worried about exercising in case it makes your pain worse?		
5 Are you worried or unhappy about taking medication for your pain?		
6 Does your back pain affect your mood and make you feel frustrated or depressed?		
7 Have you had back pain for many years?		
8 Do you have back pain at the moment?		
9 Do you have any leg pain (sciatica)?		
10 Do you have pins and needles or numbness in your legs?		
11 Do you smoke or have you ever smoked?		
12 Could your diet be healthier or more varied?		
13 Do you have difficulty passing urine?		
14 Does your pain feel worse at night?		
15 Do you have osteoporosis?		
16 Have you had any form of cancer?		

The more 'yes' answers you have, the more things you can change to have a positive effect on your health and your back pain. If you answered 'yes' to any of questions 13 to 16 you may benefit from treatment, and need to seek advice to make sure you are doing all you can to manage your back pain. This is explained in more detail below. It is likely that your fitness will have been directly affected by your back pain, and recognising this is the first step to making the changes that will improve your health and your quality of life.

Yes to questions 1 and 2:

If you think you are unfit and overweight, then you probably are! To be honest, most of us find this is the case at times, whether we have back pain or not. When you have back pain it does make it harder to exercise, but not impossible, and once you make a start it will help you manage your pain better and lose weight too. There is some evidence that losing weight alleviates back pain. Being overweight does not make you more likely to develop back pain, but being fit and having good muscle tone will certainly improve your posture, which can make you look slimmer without losing any weight at all! Part 3 includes exercises which will ease your back pain and help you back to fitness gently. To find out how to improve your posture see page 39.

weight check

Take a look at Figure 2.1 and find your height at the side and your weight along the top or bottom. Follow a line across the chart from your height until you reach the line that corresponds to your weight. Are you the right weight for your height? If not, it is time to do something about it – even small changes to your lifestyle can help you lose weight. See the healthy eating advice on page 33 and the easy-to-follow exercise programme on page 69.

Yes to question 3:

If you are off work because of your back pain it is important to think about returning. If your pain is severe and limiting your movement, it is important to have a few days off to allow you to follow the 'active rest' advice (page 49). You may need to see your GP for medication, but try over-the-counter painkillers too. If you need treatment from a physiotherapist you can arrange this privately or your GP can refer you on the NHS.

Research has shown that people who are off work for six months or more are less likely to return to work. This is not just because of pain and loss of fitness, but also the psychological issues that can arise when

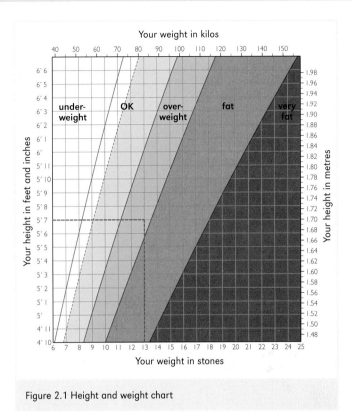

Figure 2.1 Height and weight chart

you have back pain. Many of these problems can be addressed with advice, reassurance and knowing all the facts about back pain.

Many people use back pain as an excuse to not return to a job they are unhappy in or not to do other things in their life. Be honest with yourself – if you are unhappy at work or at home think about what you need to change. A career change can be a great focus and a better motivation to get fit.

Yes to question 4:
It is normal to worry and when you are in pain it is difficult to think of anything that will help, least of all exercise. The benefits of exercise

for back pain have been known for many years, but the important thing is to pace yourself and do the right exercise for your level of pain and fitness. Part 3 includes exercises that you can use when you have severe pain and will teach you how to progress to the more active stuff when you feel ready – see the advice on 'pacing' on page 46.

Yes to question 5:

It is important to take painkillers if you need them as it will help you move more freely and get better more quickly. Many people don't like taking tablets because of worries about addiction or side-effects. In fact the risks of becoming addicted are very small if you are taking tablets correctly and for the right reasons. Side-effects are possible, but there are many different painkillers and if some don't agree with you or relieve your pain, chat to your GP or pharmacist about what else is available. On page 57 I have explained more about the different types of painkillers available.

Yes to question 6:

Many people find that they feel low or frustrated when they have back pain. Be reassured that this is a perfectly normal response to having pain and not being able to do the things you normally take for granted. If you have had back pain for a long time and think that you may be depressed, it is important not to ignore this. Confide in your GP who will be able to talk you through your options. You may choose anti-depressants, counselling or both. Improving your mood will definitely reduce the pain you are feeling. Your pain and your mood are in part a response to chemical changes in your body and taking drugs to help your pain or mood helps to bring these chemicals back into balance.

Cognitive behavioural therapy (CBT) is a type of counselling which is a good way to achieve a better understanding of your back pain, especially if you have had it for a long time. CBT has helped many people to change how they feel about back pain and how it impacts on their life. Read more about CBT on page 52.

Yes to question 7:

You may feel, if you have had your back pain for many years, that nothing has helped or can help you. I have to be honest and tell you that there isn't a cure for chronic back pain. If you have had back pain for a while, it's likely that you will have flare-ups every now and again. However, you can make the good times last longer and have shorter and fewer severe flare-ups if you exercise to improve your fitness and make a few lifestyle changes that will impact on your overall health. A history of chronic back pain places you at a higher risk of joint stiffness in your spine, and muscle weakness. A lack of exercise will make you weaker, and muscle weakness can make pain much worse. If you maintain a lifestyle which incorporates exercise, your chronic back pain will be managed much better and your acute back pain will not last as long. Read the advice on pacing (page 46) and CBT (page 52), and then give the exercises in part 3 a go.

Yes to question 8:

If this is your first episode of back pain it is important that you learn to manage your spinal health and take this as a warning that you can do more to prevent it becoming a bigger problem. See pages 56–57 for advice on how to manage your acute back pain. By strengthening your core muscles (see part 3), and improving your flexibility and posture you are less likely to have another severe episode of back pain. For advice on how to improve your posture see page 39.

Yes to question 9:

If you have sciatica, this means that one of the many nerves that supply all the joints, ligaments and muscles in your back is being irritated by inflammation, lack of movement or possibly a disc bulge nudging one of your spinal nerves. Sometimes leg pain of this kind is called 'referred pain', which means it is felt in an area away from where the problem is – the pain is in your leg, but the cause is in your back. If you have leg pain it is important that you see your GP, physiotherapist, osteopath or chiropractor for a check-up. I have included some exercises to specifically help leg pain on page 111.

Yes to question 10:

Pins and needles in the legs are common symptoms and need to be checked out. They may be a sign of nerve compression in your back. This is not something to worry about, but it needs to be monitored to make sure it doesn't get any worse as you start treatment or exercise.

Yes to question 11:

If you smoke, now is the time to stop. There are 2000 deaths every week in the UK as a result of smoking-related diseases. Smoking is a direct cause of peripheral vascular disease (narrowing of your arteries) which causes bad circulation. This will slow down your ability to heal after a flare-up of your back pain. See page 36 for information on stopping smoking.

Yes to question 12:

A healthy and balanced diet is very important for good health and maintaining a healthy weight. If you need advice on healthy eating, see page 33.

Yes to question 13:

If you have experienced problems with your bladder or going to the toilet since the onset of your back pain you must seek help immediately, as it can indicate compression of the nerve that controls your bladder and bowel. Read more about this on page 56.

Yes to question 14:

If you feel more pain in your back when you are in bed at night, you should see your GP as this could be a symptom of another illness (see page 57). He or she may also give you night-time painkillers. Sleep is an important part of your health and helps you to heal.

Yes to question 15:

If you have osteoporosis and your back pain has suddenly got much worse, it is important you see your GP or specialist for a check-up. You may have a fracture. When you are osteoporotic, fractures in the spine may result from what seem like insignificant actions. You may need a review of your medication to manage your osteoporosis better.

Yes to question 16:
If you have had cancer you will know how important it is to have regular check-ups to make sure you are in remission. Your cancer doctors or GP will arrange a check-up to establish the cause of any new or increased back pain.

Now you know your MOT results and what you need to think about, it is time to find out how you can make the lifestyle changes to improve your health and your back pain. Let's start by looking at healthy eating and stopping smoking.

healthy eating
Healthy eating is a key part of having a healthy lifestyle and managing your back pain. Eating healthily is not as hard as you may think and the benefits are well worth the effort.

If you are not eating a healthy, balanced diet, you will soon start to feel the effects and you will notice these even more as you start to exercise. Imagine driving a car: you wouldn't dream of setting off on a journey without enough fuel. A healthy diet also helps to maintain a normal body weight and can reduce your risk of developing heart disease, high blood pressure and high cholesterol. This is why you need to be aware of what kinds of food you are putting into your body, not just to feed yourself, but also as a way of keeping yourself healthy.

Drinking is just as important as eating. Most people don't drink enough and function at a level of dehydration. If you feel thirsty, it's already too late: you are dehydrated. Your body needs 2–2.5 litres of fluid a day and when you exercise you will need more. The easiest way to check how hydrated you are is to monitor the colour of your urine. It should be a pale straw colour – any darker and you're already dehydrated.

what is a healthy diet?
A healthy diet contains:

- plenty of carbohydrates or starchy foods like bread, rice, pasta, breakfast cereals, potatoes and sweet potatoes – look for higher fibre versions where possible (like wholemeal bread or pasta)
- at least five portions of a variety of fruit and vegetables daily
- moderate amounts of dairy products (or alternatives if you don't tolerate them) – look for low fat versions where possible
- moderate amounts of protein, which is found in meat, fish, eggs, beans and lentils
- the occasional treat (foods that are higher in fat, salt or added sugar should only be eaten in moderation)
- minimal salt – always read the label.

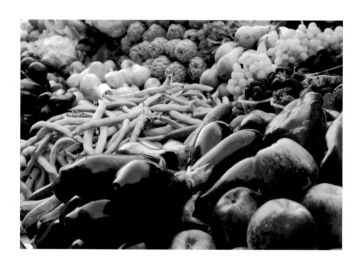

Healthy eating needn't be expensive – if you cook meals that use starchy foods and fruit and vegetables, aiming to eat less fat, salt and added sugar, it can actually work out much cheaper.

Wholegrain, high fibre foods tend to release their energy more slowly so you feel full for longer and are less likely to snack on fatty and sugary foods. Fruit and vegetables provide you with fibre that keeps your bowel healthy and also helps you feel full. Figure 2.2 shows you the different food groups and how much of each should make up your daily meals.

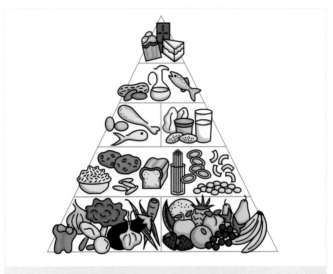

Figure 2.2 Balancing the food groups for a healthy diet

Good quantities of fresh fruit and vegetables are the way forward. Heavily processed or pre-packaged food is not only generally high in sugar but also salt and fat, all of which can contribute to weight problems, raise your cholesterol and raise your blood pressure. All of these factors will make managing your health harder.

If you need help and advice on losing weight you can join a slimming club, ask your GP to refer you to a dietician, or get advice online from the government-funded Eat Well campaign. Some useful websites are:

www.the-gi-diet.org
www.eatwell.gov.uk
www.weightwatchers.co.uk
www.dietchef.co.uk
www.slimmingworld.com

stopping smoking

One of the greatest ways to have a positive impact on your health is to stop smoking. You may be wondering what stopping smoking has to do with your back pain. Smoking affects your general health and also your circulation, and this has a direct impact on how quickly you heal and recover from injury and pain.

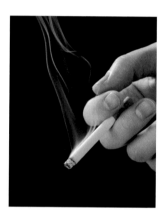

Smoking causes numerous diseases and health problems, and not just for the smoker. Both smokers and non-smokers can develop smoking-related disease. For this reason, smoking is now banned in public places and a wide range of support services has been developed to help you quit smoking.

reasons to quit

You may want to give up smoking for many reasons, from wanting to improve your health, to saving money or reducing potential harm to your family. In the UK one person dies from a smoking-related disease every four minutes. Smoking places you at a greater risk of developing heart disease, high blood pressure and peripheral vascular disease (PVD). These are some of the other diseases caused by smoking:

- lung cancer (smoking causes over 80 per cent of all lung cancer deaths)

- heart disease

- bronchitis

- strokes

- stomach ulcers

- leukaemia

- gangrene

- other cancers e.g. mouth and throat cancer.

Smoking can also make having a cold, chest problems and allergies like hay fever much worse, as well as increasing the number of wrinkles on your face and causing bad breath. It can make you cough and feel short of breath when you exercise.

> 'I really didn't believe smoking made my back pain worse! But I gave up and the improvement in my symptoms and my health has been amazing. I can even take the stairs instead of the lift at work now, without back pain and without losing my breath.'
> Jo, Yorkshire

As well as improving your own health dramatically, stopping smoking will boost your sex appeal, improve your sense of taste and smell (which will help you enjoy your healthy new diet), save you money, and protect your family's health: breathing in other people's cigarette smoke can also cause cancer. Children exposed to secondhand smoke are twice as likely to get chest problems and more likely to get ear and throat infections and asthma, while smoking during pregnancy can affect your baby's health as well as your own.

types of treatment

When willpower alone is not enough, there are various treatments and plenty of support services to help you kick the habit. Many chemists offer a 'stop smoking' service and can advise you on the products available to help you quit. There are many types of nicotine replacement therapy treatments, delivering nicotine in various ways, including gum, patches, microtabs (which dissolve under the tongue), lozenges, inhalators and nasal sprays. Other drugs that can help you to stop smoking are Zyban (bupropion hydrochloride), which changes the way that your body responds to nicotine, and Champix (varenicline), which works by reducing your craving for a cigarette and by reducing the effects you feel if you do have a cigarette. Both these treatments are only available on prescription and cannot be used if you are pregnant.

helpful contacts

Smokers are four times more likely to quit by using the NHS Stop Smoking Services together with nicotine replacement therapy than they are by using willpower alone. Find your nearest NHS service by:

- visiting the NHS Smokefree website (http://smokefree.nhs.uk) for England and Wales, or Smokeline (www.clearingtheairscotland.com) in Scotland

- texting GIVE UP and your full postcode to 88088

- telephoning the NHS Smoking Helpline (0800 022 4332) in England and Wales, or Smokeline (0800 84 84 84) in Scotland

- asking your GP or pharmacist.

The NHS Smoking Helpline in England and Wales offers free practical advice about giving up smoking, as well as a free information pack, while in Scotland, Smokeline provides free confidential advice and support. Both Smokefree and Smokeline offer an 'Ask an Expert' service.

good posture

Now you know how to help your back pain by improving your diet and stopping smoking, it is time to look at the other key things you can do to manage your back pain. One of the most important things you can improve to relieve your back pain is your posture. Making sure that you stand, sit and sleep in good positions is vital and is easy to change once you know how.

standing

Your posture is genetic to a certain extent, but you can make sure you have the best posture for you and in doing so help manage your back pain. Good posture keeps your muscles and joints in the best position to avoid the stresses and strains which can cause aching and pain. Don't be put off by the fact that when you first start to stand and sit well your postural muscles can ache, especially if they haven't been used for a while.

> ### standing – key points
> - Know your postural type
> - Know how to manage your postural type
> - Stay fit and strong.

If you know your postural type, it is easier to manage it and strengthen and stretch where your muscles are weak or tight. Figure 2.3 shows the main postural types – all variations of normal – and how they affect your muscles. If you look at yourself in a full-length mirror wearing just your underwear or tight clothing, you will be able to compare your posture with the four diagrams. The other option is to take a photograph of

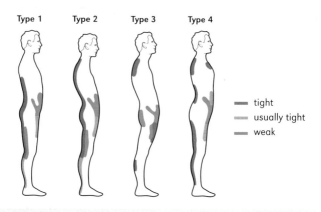

Figure 2.3 The main postural types

yourself side-on and compare it to the diagram. You can get a friend to do this for you or photograph your reflection in the mirror.

- **Type 1:** This shows an increased lumbar (low back) curve and puts strain on the small facet joints (see page 10) of the lumbar spine because it is bent too far backwards. If you have this posture, see pages 96 and 100–101 to learn which exercise will help you make your spine stronger.

- **Type 2:** This posture has an excessive range in two of the curves in your spine. It places strain on the lumbar spine because it is bent too far backwards, and on the thoracic spine (mid back) as it is bent too far forwards and rounded at the shoulders. This is a very common posture if you sit at a desk all day. The exercises on page 112 will help this postural type.

- **Type 3:** This is a classic lazy posture which relies on your ligaments rather than your muscles. Strain tends to be felt at the top of the lumbar spine as this is where most of the movement occurs, especially when you bend backwards. For exercises to help see pages 104–107.

- **Type 4:** This is the opposite of posture type 2 above and has a reduction of both spinal curves. Again, this influences the way the muscles that support your spine work. It is common in people who do or have done lots of sport and don't stretch. For exercises to help see pages 106–107.

Once you know the areas where you are likely to be weak or tight you can start to exercise and stretch to target specific muscles and joints, and really change your back pain.

lifting

Many people blame lifting heavy items for having started their back pain. Just because you have a bad back doesn't mean you can't lift: it is easy to learn safe and correct lifting technique and avoid the recurrence of back pain and injury.

The strongest muscles to help you lift are in your legs. By bending your knees and getting as close as you can to what you are lifting, you are putting yourself in the best position to lift. Using the powerful leg muscles to bring you back into a standing position avoids straining the muscles in the back.

If you are having problems with lifting at work, ask for lifting and handling training. Your employer has a legal responsibility to arrange this for you. If you are a carer, speak to your doctor, who will be able to advise you who can help teach you to lift and handle safely.

Lifting – key points
- Bend your knees to lift and lower, not your waist
- Keep your back straight
- Keep what you are lifting as close to you as possible
- Stand up with your head first
- Turn with your feet and not your body when lifting or carrying
- Keep your feet wide apart and when possible one in front of the other so you are more stable and less likely to twist.

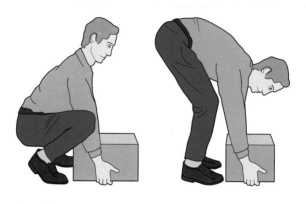

Figure 2.4 Lifting – right and wrong

Figure 2.4 shows the difference between bad and good lifting technique and how you can use your legs to protect your spine.

sitting

We all spend much of our day sitting at work, in the car and at home. It is easy to cause stress and strain to the spine and overstretch the muscles and ligaments by sitting incorrectly. This alone can cause aching and pain.

To demonstrate this, take your little finger, bend it backwards, and hold it there for two minutes. When you release your finger you will feel an ache and stiffness that is similar to the ache you may feel after sitting for too long. You wouldn't dream of keeping your finger in that position for any longer than the two minutes, but you will regularly do this to your spine, by sitting for hours at a time at your computer or in the car.

> **TIP**
> Put your socks and trousers on while sitting down. Don't try to balance on one leg when you are in pain.

The best way to avoid this kind of back pain is to get up and walk around, and stretch every hour or so. At work, use your lunch break to walk to a shop to buy your lunch or take a short walk after you have eaten – this also builds some exercise into your day. Regularly changing your posture while sitting (see box) to give your spine a rest is also easy to do. Remember, there is no perfect posture if you remain in it for too long. This doesn't only apply to the lower back. Think about how you use your phone – whether you're leaning or reaching to one side or, the very worst, holding the phone to your shoulder with your ear! If you are doing this on a regular basis at work ask for a headset to help avoid back and neck pain.

> ## Sitting – key points
> - Don't sit in the same position for too long
> - Get up and move around at least every hour
> - Take a walk in your lunch hour to stretch out all your muscles
> - While sitting at your desk, do some simple postural exercises – slumping, tipping your pelvis and squeezing your buttocks – to relieve muscle pain in your back and neck
> - Look at how you use your phone – a headset can help
> - Look at how your chair and desk are set up – simple changes can minimise strain on your back.

Figure 2.5 shows how your work station should be set up to support your back. The type of chair you have and how you adjust it to make it fit your body are essential. You can have the best chair in the world, but if you don't adjust it to suit you, you may as well sit on a bad chair. If you are concerned about your work station ask your HR department to arrange a personal ergonomic assessment which will recommend what you need to improve your posture.

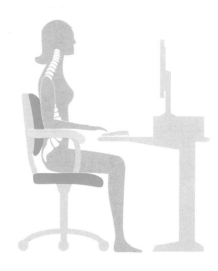

Figure 2.5 A well-designed work station

WORK STATION TIPS

- Use an adjustable height computer monitor, or rest the monitor on books if necessary to raise it up to eye level.
- Make sure you have a chair with armrests, and adjust them to support your elbows.
- Arrange your desk to make sure you don't have to reach repeatedly for items such as the phone.
- Make sure your thighs are fully supported by the seat of the chair.
- Don't sit with your legs crossed – keep your feet flat on the floor or on a foot rest to support them
- Make sure your hips and knees are at 90 degrees.
- Ask for a chair that can be adjusted to support your lower back.

sleeping

How you sleep is just as important as how you sit. If you sleep eight hours per night you will spend 56 hours per week, 224 hours over four weeks and 2912 hours per year in bed! This is a lot of hours to put your back under stress. Your mattress and pillow need to support your spine in a neutral posture which ensures it is not unduly bent or twisted. Figure 2.6 shows how the spine should be supported by your mattress and how it can be vulnerable if your mattress is too hard or too soft for your posture and flexibility.

> **TIP**
> To get out of bed roll onto your side, and use your hands and elbow to push yourself up into sitting position. The weight of your legs sliding off the bed will also help. You will find this much easier and it won't hurt as much.

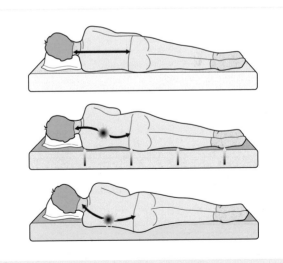

Figure 2.6 Good sleeping posture (top)

You don't need to spend a lot of money on an expensive bed, but do take the time to find the right one for you. Price is not always the best indicator. Comfort is the most important consideration, not whether or not it is an 'orthopaedic bed' or made from special 'memory foam'. Another back pain myth is that you should sleep on the floor or a hard board – this is not recommended to alleviate back pain, nor is it conducive to a good night's sleep!

A good rule of thumb is to buy a mattress with 1000-plus pocket springs. The more you have the better, as they will provide your back with more support and you can choose whether they are firm, medium or soft. This is always down to personal preference. Try as many types of mattress as possible and with your partner, if you share your bed, and don't rush the decision.

> **TIP**
> Loosen your back with gentle exercise before you get out of bed in the morning. See page 104 for examples.

● pacing yourself

Pacing yourself is one of the most important concepts to practise and will help you stop doing either too much or too little, both of which are very common when you have back pain. Here are two common scenarios which you may recognise.

- **Overdoing it**
  You are not in pain, so you run around getting all the jobs done that you haven't been able to do because of previous back pain. Because you feel good, you keep going, happily ticking things off your list. As you carry on you feel increasing pain until you can't keep it up and you have to rest. Unfortunately the pain is worse after your rest and worse still the next day, sometimes for two or three days. As the cycle continues, you have to rest for longer periods, putting you off doing the activity again. You lose fitness, and become frustrated and depressed.

- **Underdoing it**
  You are in pain and only get relief when you rest. You have had to stop working as a result of your pain and now spend much of your time resting, unable to go out or to the gym. Your family are supportive and do your shopping for you or run errands. You have become unfit and have put on weight, but can't do anything about it because of your pain. You may lose confidence, start to feel that you don't have a role within the workplace or family, and may feel depressed and have difficulty sleeping.

returning to work

The average amount of time taken off work for each episode of back pain is 19 days. The cost of this to business is huge, but this doesn't take into account the emotional and personal cost to you. Taking responsibility for your back through simple, sensible precautions at work and at home can reduce the misery of back pain and how it impacts on your life. Long-term sickness is not appropriate for back pain. If necessary, seriously consider changing your job to allow you this flexibility. For further information check out these websites:

- www.betterbacks.hse.gov.uk
- www.backinaction.co.uk
- www.realhealth.org.uk

Both of these are common ways that people try to manage their back pain. Unfortunately, neither is effective and in the long run the pain and disability increase. Learning how to pace yourself can be hard, but if you follow these four easy steps you will be able to use the pacing principle in all areas of your life.

step 1: measure your activity

You probably have very little idea how long it takes you to perform various tasks before you start to experience pain. To control your pain, you need to know how long you can continue with a task or activity before your pain will increase. The key to this is to time yourself and work out how many minutes it takes to bring on your pain.

step 2: set yourself a limit

To set yourself a limit, take the time you measured and take off 20 per cent. This is your limit. For example, if your pain comes on after 10 minutes of ironing your limit is 8 minutes. You must not go over your limit: use a timer to make you stop.

step 3: stick to the limit

This is the hard bit – when the timer says stop, go and do something else or rest. How long for is for you to decide – it may vary from a few minutes if you have been ironing to a few days if you were gardening. The idea is to find your happy medium. It may be frustrating but I guarantee it will work.

step 4: increase your limit

Once you know your limit and you can stick to it and get the job done without increasing your pain, it is time to increase your limit. Decide before you start how much more time you will allow and only increase gradually. Jumping from 8 minutes of housework to 30 minutes is likely to be too much too soon – 15 minutes may be more realistic and keep you active and pain free.

In time you will see an increase in what you are able to do without pain. It often helps to keep a record, so that you can look back and see how far you have come.

'Patience, acceptance and exercise are the three most important things that having back pain has taught me. I thought I would never get better, but I did – it just took longer than I thought it would. I still get back pain, but I know how to pace myself and manage it much better now.'

Rob, London

use pacing to increase:

- how long you can spend doing housework
- how long you can spend gardening
- how long you can stay at work when you first go back
- how many days a week you can work when you first go back
- how long you can exercise or how many exercises you can do
- how long you can drive before you need to get out and stretch.

active rest

In the past it was thought that bed rest was the best thing for a bad back, but it is now known that this is not the case. Research over a number of years has shown that rest is not helpful for treating back pain, and may even be a factor in making pain and fitness worse. The more active you can be while respecting your pain the better. This is what is called 'active rest'.

> 'Don't stay in bed, keep moving, is the best advice I ever had. You don't always feel like it, but it's so much better than letting your muscles waste. That just means more time in the gym getting the strength back again.'
>
> Jane, London

You may need a few days off work when your back pain is severe – but this does not mean you need to stay in bed. It is important to remain active around the house, get dressed, take short walks, have short rests and do exercises advised by your physiotherapist or those featured in this book. Consider working part-time if your symptoms are severe: this allows you to stay at work while being realistic about needing time to allow pain to settle. GPs now issue 'fit to work' notes rather than sick notes, to inform employers about the importance of returning part-time and pacing an increase in activity, rather than encouraging people to be off work for extended periods.

● what help can I get?

Many people can help you manage your back pain. It is unlikely that you will need the services of all these professionals, as self-management is the most important part of managing back pain, but it doesn't hurt to know who they are.

Your GP and other practitioners can provide valuable advice and information but there is always more than one treatment plan, as what works best for one person won't necessarily work best for you. Talking about the different treatment options available will help you create and choose a plan that is right for you and your lifestyle.

the physiotherapist/osteopath/chiropractor

Physiotherapy sees full and functional movement at the heart of what it means to be healthy. Working with a physiotherapist will allow you to develop, maintain and restore movement to your spine during and after a flare-up of back pain, help you manage your pain and prevent further issues and movement problems.

finding a practitioner
Physiotherapists: Your GP can refer you to a physiotherapist on the NHS or privately. You can also find your own private physiotherapist via the internet, word of mouth or the phone book. Make sure they are a chartered physiotherapist and have the letters MCSP (Member of the Chartered Society of Physiotherapy) or HPC (Health Professions Council) after their name as this will ensure they are fully approved and qualified. If they work in the NHS they will definitely be chartered.

Osteopaths: Osteopaths should be registered with the General Osteopathic Council which ensures that they are fully qualified and licensed to practice. Check that they are registered before you book to see them. Most osteopaths practice privately and you can refer yourself for treatment. Some work in the NHS and you can be referred by your GP. This varies depending on where you live and if the service is available on the NHS. Look on the internet or in the phone book to find a local practitioner.

Chiropractors: Chiropractors should be registered with the General Chiropractic Council. Again they practice privately and you can find details for local practitioners on the internet or in the phone book.

All practitioners need an initial appointment to assess you fully. Be prepared to undress to your underwear, or take a pair of shorts if this will make you feel more comfortable. This appointment may last up to 45 minutes, but further treatment sessions will probably be shorter. Every practitioner will work differently and may see you on a weekly basis until you improve or feel able to manage your back pain yourself with exercises and stretches.

TIP

Ask to be referred to a physiotherapist for advice, but start by managing what you can on your own. Arrange treatment if required but remember back pain is best managed by you.

the pharmacist

Your high street pharmacist is the best person to advise you on which medications can help you without a prescription. Use the same pharmacist for all your prescription and non-prescription drugs as they can then monitor what you take and check for any interactions between drugs, supplements and alternative therapies.

NHS Direct
This is a useful source of advice if you are concerned and are unable to see your GP. It can help you make a decision on the most appropriate management for your back pain, and advise you who you should see if things become worse. The number for NHS Direct is 0845 46 47.

the dietician
If you have back pain it is easy to overeat as exercise may be limited. Simple advice can have a major impact on your weight and consequently your pain. A dietician can advise you on foods that can help boost the immune system, and help you ensure you are getting enough of the right vitamins and minerals in your diet to help keep your body strong and healthy to deal with any medication or pain.

the pain management team
If you have had back pain for a long time and are unable to control your pain, your doctor may refer you to the specialist pain management team at your local hospital. Such teams can offer alternative medications, treatments and exercise programmes to help you manage your pain better. They use cognitive behavioural therapy (see below) as a basis for the treatment they offer, which is aimed at helping you to help yourself.

cognitive behavioural therapy (CBT)
Medications and other treatments may be a key part of managing your back pain, but successful treatment depends just as much on your attitude and your emotional health. Your ability to cope despite pain often determines how much of an impact it will have on your day-to-day life. Studies show that people who take control of their treatment and actively manage their back pain experience less pain and function better.

CBT is a way of talking about how you think about yourself, how you relate to the world, and how what you do affects your thoughts and feelings. In relation to back pain, it can help you focus on the problems and difficulties you are having, instead of on the causes of your distress or symptoms. One of the ways it works is by breaking problems down into smaller parts, making it easier to see how many things – your thoughts, emotions, physical feelings and actions – relate to your back pain.

All these things are closely linked, and how you think about your pain can affect how you feel physically and emotionally. It can also alter what you do about your back pain.

> 'I believed for years someone else could and would fix my back and I spent a fortune on treatments and so-called cures. When I met a therapist who told me it was only me who could fix my back I didn't want to believe it. But she was right, and now I understand the facts, and how pacing and taking responsibility for my own health makes all the difference. I still get pain, but I cope with it better than I did. I'm thinner, fitter and I'm also richer as I stopped wasting my money looking for a cure and a quick fix.'
>
> Brian, London

CBT can be done individually, in a group, or even via the internet or by using a self-help book. If you see a therapist, you will usually have sessions lasting between 30 and 60 minutes, and after discussing your past life and background you will agree on short, medium and long term goals. Over the period of treatment – probably between six weeks and six months – you will look at your thoughts, feelings and behaviours to work out whether they are unrealistic or unhelpful, how they interact and how they affect you. The therapist will then help you to work out how to change unhelpful thoughts and behaviours.

The availability of CBT varies between different areas and there may be a waiting list for treatment. Your GP can refer you. The beauty of CBT is that you can continue to develop your skills by yourself even after your sessions have finished.

information on CBT
For further information see the CBT web pages of PsychNet-UK (www.psychnet-uk.com/psychotherapy/psychotherapy_cognitive_behavioural_therapy.htm) and the Royal College of Psychiatrists (www.rcpsych.ac.uk/mentalhealthinfoforall.aspx). Other useful websites are:

- www.babcp.com (British Association for Behavioural and Cognitive Psychotherapies)
- http://moodgym.anu.edu.au (information, quizzes, games and skills training to help prevent depression and low mood)
- www.livinglifetothefull.com (free online life skills courses)

complementary therapists
People who aren't helped by painkillers or don't like taking tablets sometimes turn to complementary and alternative medicine. This includes homeopathy, magnets, supplements and acupuncture. Few of these treatments have been extensively studied in clinical trials, so it is difficult to assess whether complementary therapies are helpful for back pain. If you are interested in trying complementary and alternative therapy discuss it with your doctor or physiotherapist. They will be able to help you decide if it's right for you, and will save you a considerable amount of money if it is unlikely to help you.

acupuncture
This uses tiny needles, which are inserted into your skin at precise points on the body. It is believed that the needles stimulate the body's energy channels and this helps to relieve pain. It is also believed that putting the needle into the skin stimulates the immune system to release pain-relieving chemicals in the body. Studies of acupuncture for back pain have been mixed, but most have found some short-term relief

of pain. From my experience, I find it very useful to reduce muscle spasm and pain.

Acupuncture is safe if you select a reputable practitioner, and physiotherapists and doctors are often trained to practise it. All physiotherapists who practise acupuncture should be registered with the AACP (Acupuncture Association of Chartered Physiotherapists) and can be found via their website, www.aacp.org.uk. Doctors who practise acupuncture will be registered with the BMAS (British Medical Acupuncture Society) and can be found at www.medical-acupuncture.co.uk.

'Acupuncture really helps me when my back flares up. It's not a cure, but it means I can move and stop myself getting stiff. It also means I can stay at work and keep exercising. I don't have time for back pain! I have to live my life – sometimes it just has to be a little slower than I like.'

David, London

● the surgeon

Surgery is only required in 5 per cent of cases of back pain, and if pain is your main symptom, can be avoided if you have good self-management alongside conservative treatments such as good posture, physiotherapy, and spinal stability exercises. Surgery to manage pain is most helpful if you have severe leg pain (sciatica) that does not ease, rather than back pain. It is otherwise only useful if you have symptoms that indicate nerve compression or cauda equina syndrome (see page 19).

● surgery for back pain

Surgery for back pain is generally reserved for those who suffer neurological symptoms that are at risk of becoming worse, or severe pain that isn't relieved by other treatments. Surgical treatments include:

- **Discectomy:** this operation is performed on herniated discs that are pressing on a nerve root in the spine, and causing severe leg pain and serious neurological symptoms.
- **Decompression:** this kind of surgery can be beneficial if you suffer from spinal stenosis, causing narrowing of the central or lateral canal where the nerve root sits.
- **Fusion:** surgeons can also permanently fuse joints in the spine to increase stability and reduce pain.
- **Disc replacement:** this is a fairly new procedure that is effective for some (though not all) people with degenerative disc disease. The central part of the disc (the nucleus) is the part which is replaced with gel, ceramic or metal to restore shock absorbency and space between the vertebrae.

● acute pain: know the warning signs

When you know the warning signs that need medical attention you can reassure yourself that nothing serious is wrong, even when you have severe back pain. Signs to look out for are:

- **Bladder or bowel problems:** Being unable to pass urine is called urinary retention and is an acute and urgent problem that needs full investigation. It could indicate compression of the cauda equina (see page 19) and you should go to A&E.
- **Unexplained weight loss and feeling unwell:** This could be due to another illness and your back pain may or may not be linked. Go to your GP who can investigate fully.

- **Night pain:** Pain can feel worse at night because you are not distracted with work and chores. This can make you more anxious, but it may simply be due to lying in one position too long and muscle spasm making it difficult to move easily. However, see your GP if your sleep is disturbed and you are unable to lie down because your pain is worse than during the day.
- **Loss of sensation and weakness in one or both legs:** This may indicate irritation or compression of a nerve in the back. It requires assessment to find out how serious the problem is. See your physiotherapist or GP who can assess you and arrange to get you treated appropriately.
- **Severe leg pain:** This may indicate that a nerve root in your back is inflamed or compressed. A physiotherapist can check for weakness, and teach you how to sit more comfortably and give you specific exercises to help manage the pain. Your GP can prescribe medication to help manage nerve pain and refer you to a physiotherapist.

> **TIP**
> Know which drugs work for you, either over the counter or on prescription, and make sure you have them readily available at home for when you need them.

pain control and medication

Pain that persists despite initial treatment may require medication. Don't assume that taking medication is all you need to do to get the most from your treatment – you should continue exercising when possible and resting when necessary. Continue trying to lose weight if you need to.

Taking medication regularly instead of waiting for pain to increase will lessen the overall intensity of your discomfort. Many people hate taking medication but it is an essential part of managing your symptoms. There will come a time when you can reduce your medication. Think about it another way: if your drugs control your back pain and allow you to exercise, this will reduce your pain further, which allows you to take less medication.

⬤ NSAIDs and other painkillers

- Standard painkillers like paracetamol and anti-inflammatories like ibuprofen will help. Your pharmacist can advise you about other over-the-counter drugs that may help.

- Non-steroidal anti-inflammatory drugs (NSAIDs) are the most commonly prescribed and widely used drugs. They can relieve pain and reduce inflammation. Over-the-counter NSAIDs include ibuprofen, but stronger NSAIDs are available on prescription. NSAIDs have risks of side-effects that increase when used at high dosages for long-term treatment, including gastric ulcers, cardio-vascular problems, gastrointestinal bleeding, and liver and kidney damage. Consuming alcohol or taking corticosteroids while using NSAIDs regularly also increases your risk of gastrointestinal bleeding.

⬤ other prescription medication

If you have tried other treatments but are still experiencing severe pain and disability, you and your doctor can discuss other treatments. Stronger prescription analgesics (pain relieving drugs) are available – although unlike NSAIDs these do not relieve inflammation – including:

- Tramadol: this acts on the central nervous system to reduce your pain, and can provide effective pain relief with fewer side effects than NSAIDs though it may cause nausea, drowsiness and consti-pation. It is generally used for short-term treatment of acute pain.

- Prescription painkillers such as codeine may provide relief from more severe pain like that caused by arthritis in the spine. These stronger medications can be addictive but the risk is thought to be small in people who have severe pain. Side-effects may include nausea, constipation and drowsiness.

> 'I hate taking painkillers and I was afraid of the side-effects and causing more damage if I couldn't feel the pain. But if I use them when my pain is at its worst it allows me to keep active, which means I don't have to take them for as long. I now realise that pain doesn't always mean damage and movement really does help.'
>
> Ed, London

- Amytriptoline: again this works in the central nervous system and is used to treat nerve pain. It is very effective in treating leg pain caused by pressure on a nerve root in your spine.

⬤ facet joint and epidural injections

These injections are offered as an option when treatments such as physiotherapy, manual therapies, acupuncture, prescription drugs and time have failed to improve your symptoms. Your GP will need to refer you to a specialist for this type of treatment, which is available both on the NHS and privately.

- **Injections of corticosteroid** into your spinal joints can be helpful in treating some types of back pain. Steroids are potent drugs which can reduce swelling and inflammation quickly. However, your doctor may limit the number of injections you can have each year, since too many steroid injections may cause joint damage.

- **Epidurals** are injections into the spinal canal and can be effective for severe leg pain. They don't work for everyone and can have side-effects but your doctor may offer you this as a treatment option. These are different from the epidurals you might have to give birth, which make you numb from the waist down.

The NICE guidelines now state that the use of injection therapy is not helpful as a treatment for non-specific mechanical low back pain. Injections are more helpful in the treatment of leg pain if a nerve root in the spine is inflamed or compressed.

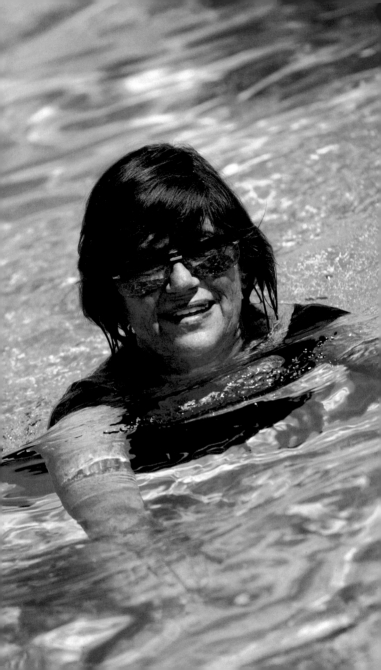

part 3

the exercises

where do I start?

You have already made an important first step in changing the way you manage your back pain by reading this book. Ask your doctor for a referral to a physiotherapist or the local leisure centre for exercise on prescription if you want help to get started. They can help you create a personal, well-paced exercise plan that will strengthen the muscles that support your spine, increase your range of movement and reduce your pain. This may be the confidence boost you need to support the self-management advice in this book.

The next thing to consider once you have decided to use exercise to manage your pain and your fitness is where to start. I will show you how to return to exercise with confidence. There are so many myths about exercise and back pain it's a wonder anyone believes anything any more! Everyone has heard the 'no pain, no gain' theory, but this will do little to encourage you to exercise and get back to fitness. Exercise doesn't have to hurt, and physical pain can be avoided if you exercise within your ability. You should expect muscular aches, as this is normal after exercise, but increased back pain can be avoided.

When you have back pain, regular, gentle exercise can help by increasing circulation and reducing spasm. If you have been inactive for a while, you need to start with less strenuous activities such as walking or swimming to get your fitness back. There is an introductory walking plan in this book (page 83) and a section about exercising in water (see page 77). Beginning at a slow pace will allow you to become fitter without straining yourself. As you become fitter, you will be able to do more. On page 78 you will find exercises to do specifically when you have back pain. As you read on you will find more specific exercises to strengthen your core, buttocks and legs, and improve your balance.

Your personality and experience of exercise will influence how you react, and this part of the book will help you choose the right exercises and lifestyle changes for you to manage your pain, and get fitter along the way.

the benefits of exercise

Regular exercise can not only help your back pain but will help you to:

- reduce the risk of dying prematurely from heart disease
- reduce the risk of developing diabetes
- reduce the risk of developing high blood pressure
- reduce high blood pressure if you already have it
- reduce feelings of depression and anxiety
- control your weight
- reduce the risk of osteoporosis
- build and maintain healthy bones, muscles and joints
- improve balance and reduce the risk of falling.

For the greatest overall benefits, it is recommended that you do 20 to 30 minutes of aerobic activity three or more times a week, and some type of muscle strengthening activity, as well as stretching, twice a week. If you are unable to do this because of your back pain, you can still gain substantial benefits by accumulating 30 minutes of moderate-intensity exercise every day. This can be as simple as walking to and from work or the shops, hoovering, climbing the stairs or even cleaning. It is important to remember that when you have back pain you may not be able to do as much. Little and often will still make a difference.

'Back pain took over my life for a while but knowing what to expect as I improved, coming off my medication and accepting that there is no magic pill or quick fix, made it easier for me to get back to work and back to the gym.'

Sandra, Scotland

before you start

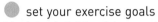 set your exercise goals

It's always helpful to have a goal – it helps keep you motivated and makes you think twice about skipping an exercise session! If you are exercising for the first time since your back pain started, make sure you choose something that is achievable. It may be as simple as walking every day, or doing one of the acute pain exercises on pages 104–107. It is also important to consider a variety of forms of exercise that will help you. This stops you getting bored, and some types of exercise may be easier than others when you have acute back pain and muscle spasm.

exercise and back pain – key points

- Start gently and increase the intensity of your exercise programme gradually.
- Cool down after exercise with gentle stretches (see pages 75–76 for ideas).
- Pay attention to good technique and try to move smoothly.
- Don't force your back beyond a comfortable range of motion – the range will increase the more you exercise.
- If your back feels particularly painful afterwards, reduce the intensity of your next exercise session.
- If an activity causes you pain or increases your pain beyond what is normal then stop.
- Increase incidental activity in your lifestyle. For example, walk to the nearby shops instead of driving.

gym or home?

You may be surprised how much exercise you can do at home: you don't need to build an extension for your own gym or to buy expensive gym equipment. You can easily do most of the exercises in this book at home with little or no equipment. A gym ball (see page 91) is helpful for exercises and stretching, but you can manage without one.

⚫ medication and medical conditions

If you have any other diagnosed medical conditions it doesn't mean you can't exercise. However, check with your doctor that you are not going to do yourself any harm. Most medical conditions will benefit from exercise, whether they are related to your mental or physical health – you may just need to be monitored until your level of fitness improves. If you are taking medication that affects your metabolism (for example with diabetes and thyroid problems) you may need to monitor the effect of exercise until you get used to training. Again, if you have any concerns chat to your doctor.

⚫ pregnancy and post-natal back pain

If you are currently pregnant and used to exercising, carry on as long as you feel well enough to do so. Exercise will help your back pain and keep you fit for the delivery. As you get bigger you may find it less comfortable but you can still exercise.

If you have just had a baby and are suffering from back pain, it is important to have your post-natal checks. You need to make sure your tummy muscles are recovering and that you are doing your pelvic floor exercises. A good bra is even more important at this time. If you are breastfeeding get measured for a sports bra from a good department store or specialist bra shop, and try to get measured when your breasts are at their fullest. A second 'pull over' soft bra or sports top with a built in bra/crop top will provide more support, and allow for any fluctuation in size. For further advice visit www.lessbounce.co.uk or www.bravissimo.com.

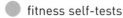 fitness self-tests

It is important not to overestimate your current level of fitness. Be honest with yourself and you will ensure that you start at the right place for you and progress quickly without any setbacks due to pain or illness. If you are an experienced exerciser looking to increase the amount of training you are doing, it is just as important to be as realistic as a complete beginner. Doing too much too soon will make your back pain worse. Even when you are feeling at your fittest, make sure you pace yourself (see page 46) and listen to your body.

These quick and simple self-tests will allow you to map your progress every four to six weeks. Prepare to be amazed by how much you can improve in the first six weeks. This is really important if you have chronic back pain as it can be hard to stay motivated at times. This will also help with pacing yourself and knowing your own limits.

preparing to exercise at home

Exercising at home needs minimal preparation – put aside some time every day, or grab a spare five minutes when you can.

- Clear a space – move the coffee table or anything you could trip over out of the way.
- Wear comfortable clothes and supportive shoes – trainers are best.
- Make sure the room isn't too hot – open a window.
- Have some water to hand in case you get thirsty.
- Stick some motivating music on, and get moving.
- Make sure you won't be interrupted, and turn off your mobile phone!

All these tests are simple and easy to do. Set an alarm for one minute and do as many repetitions as you can. Make a note of how many repetitions you have managed each time you do the tests.

step-ups

- Use any step. If you don't have stairs at home you could use the kerb at the side of the road.
- Use the banister or wall for balance if you need to.
- Step up with your right foot first, ensuring your whole foot is on the step, then bring the left foot up beside it.
- Step down with your right leg, bringing the left foot to join it.
- Repeat, leading with your left leg.

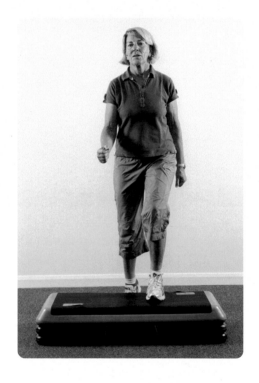

press-ups (against a wall, bench, or kitchen worktop depending how fit you are!)

- Place your hands shoulder width apart on the surface of your choice.
- Step your feet away from the surface and rest your weight through your hands.
- Slowly bend your elbows and lower your chest towards the wall/surface.
- Then push yourself away from the wall/surface.
- Make sure you don't arch your back.

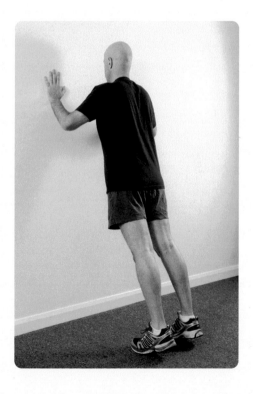

squats

- Stand with your feet hip distance apart.
- Bend your knees as far as you comfortably can, as if you are going to sit down.
- Keep your knees behind your toes and stick your bottom out behind you.

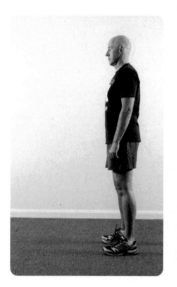 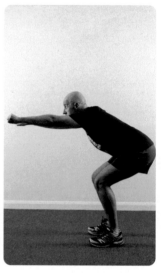

If you prefer, you can use walking as a way of seeing how much you have improved. Time yourself walking a set distance (count the number of times you need to rest). Soon you will be able to walk the distance without a rest.

Alternatively, pick any exercise from later in this book and count the number of repetitions you can do in one minute. Remember to rest as many times as you need to. The rest breaks will reduce as your fitness improves.

getting back to fitness: home routine

This set of exercise ideas is designed to help you return to fitness, perhaps if you have been off work with back pain, and will complement the specific strengthening exercises and stretches that are outlined later in this book. This simple routine – I don't like to call it a programme as it is not intended to be that regimented – will build up noticeable pace and stamina in only a few weeks. Try doing the full routine (steps 1–9) three times a week, and you will be impressed with your results. However, the exercises can be mixed and matched to make up a personal routine, so if one exercise causes you pain, substitute another. Remember that this book aims to help you manage your back pain.

Once this routine becomes easy, progress to the walking or swimming programmes (pages 83 and 78) and see your fitness improve even more.

warm-up and stretching

march on the spot

1 March on the spot to warm up. Start at a moderate pace that you can maintain for the full 2–6 minutes. Swing your arms and lift your knees high. You should aim to become breathless but still be able to talk easily.

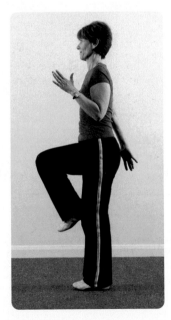

- week 1: march for 2 minutes
- week 2: march for 4 minutes
- week 3: march for 6 minutes

squats

2   Stand with your feet hip distance apart and your hands by
your sides. Squat as if to sit down, and then stand tall,
reaching your arms out in front. Lift your arms alternately and feel
the stretch in your side.

- week 1: sit to stand 5 times
- week 2: sit to stand 10 times
- week 3: sit to stand 15 times

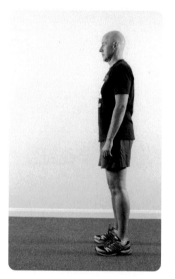 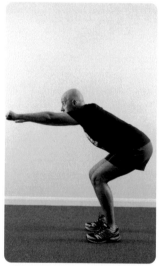

step back lunge

3 Stand with your feet hip distance apart and your hands on your hips. Step back with one leg, as far as you would if you were walking backwards, then return it to the starting position. Repeat 5–15 times, holding the final step back and keeping your heel on the floor. Hold for 30 seconds, then repeat with the other leg. You will feel the stretch in the back of your leg.

- week 1: step back 5 times
- week 2: step back 10 times
- week 3: step back 15 times

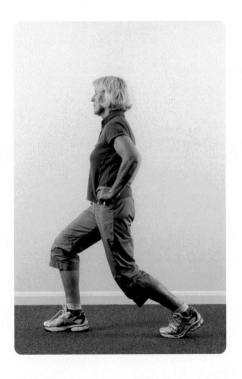

aerobic exercises

As you improve you can add aerobic exercise, which will increase your heart rate and fat burning.

step-ups

4 Step-ups can be performed on a small box or at the bottom of your staircase. Step up and down with one leg 5–15 times and then change legs. This is one 'set' or repetition. Continue for 2–6 sets with one minute's rest between each set. Maintain a good posture by standing up tall with your shoulders back, looking straight ahead, and keep sipping water between sets so you do not dehydrate.

- week 1: step up 5 times for 2 sets
- week 2: step up 10 times for 4 sets
- week 3: step up 15 times for 6 sets

bicep curl and press

5 Strengthening your arms with bicep curls and an overhead press will help improve your overall strength and posture. Hold a weight in each hand (see box on page 74), starting with 0.4–2 kg weights depending on your level of fitness. Stand tall and alternate your arms, bending your arm from your side to your shoulder then pushing the weight above your head. Repeat 5–15 times for one set. Continue for 2 to 4 sets with a minute's rest between sets.

- week 1: lift 5 times for 2 sets
- week 2: lift 10 times for 3 sets
- week 3: lift 15 times for 4 sets

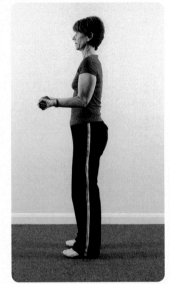

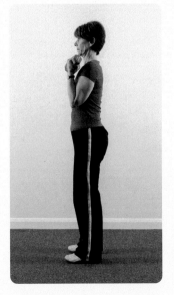

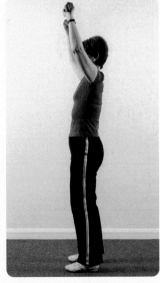

weights

You don't have to buy expensive weights: you can use tins of beans (400 g) or bags of sugar (1 kg) as weights in each hand. If you want to buy weights, start with light weights and progress as you become stronger. You can buy beginner's sets of 1–5 kg weights from most sports stores, but don't try to lift too much too soon.

side bends

6 Using your home-made weights in each hand, keep your arms by your sides. Slowly lean over to the right, allowing your hand to reach your mid-thigh. Bring the other arm up and over your head. Repeat 5–15 times and then repeat on the left side. This is one set. After one minute's rest continue for 2–6 sets.

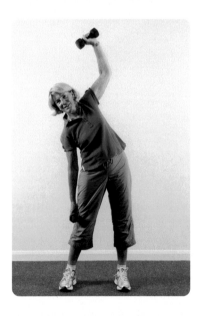

- week 1: bend to each side 5 times for 2 sets
- week 2: bend to each side 10 times for 4 sets
- week 3: bend to each side 15 times for 6 sets

winding down and toning stretches

7 March on the spot slowly, concentrating on your posture and lifting your knees. Breathe deeply in and out, keeping your hands on your waist. This will allow your heart rate to return to normal as you keep moving and allow your body to cool down gradually.

- week 1: march for 2 minutes
- week 2: march for 4 minutes
- week 3: march for 6 minutes

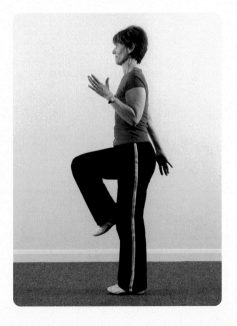

8 Stand with your hands resting on a kitchen surface or the back of a steady chair. Lift one leg out behind you, making sure you don't arch your back, and lift the foot off the floor. Squeeze your bottom as you lift. Repeat 5–15 times and then change legs.

- week 1: lift each leg back 5 times
- week 2: lift each leg back 10 times
- week 3: lift each leg back 15 times

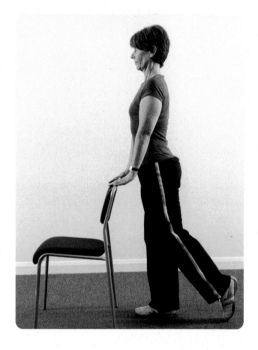

9 Stand up straight, and take six deep breaths in through your nose. Breathe out through your mouth, making sure you empty your lungs, and gently lift your pelvic floor (see page 98). You will feel your lower tummy gently tighten as you do this, working your core muscles which protect the spine.

getting back to fitness: swimming

Your local swimming pool is a great place to start exercising if you have back pain. Because your body weight is supported, swimming enables you to move more easily and reduce muscle spasm. This will allow you to restore normal movement more quickly and reduce your pain.

Exercising for just 12 weeks is all it takes to start seeing results such as:

- increased muscle strength

- improved mood and quality of sleep

- reduced fear of exercise

- greater flexibility

- loss of excess body fat

- reduced risk of exercise-related injuries.

Your weight is 'reduced' by up to 90 per cent in water and swimming can give you the buoyancy you need to keep you exercising aerobically for longer than on dry land. This is a bonus if you need to lose weight. Swimming is an excellent exercise which increases your heart rate, with an added benefit over walking as it exercises both the upper and lower body at the same time.

As with any new exercise, you must monitor the effects on your back pain and take the necessary action to pace yourself. Before you start:

- Always check with your doctor that swimming is advisable for you.

- Check that the pool is easy to access – if you are in pain, how difficult is it to get in and out of the pool?

aqua aerobics

An aqua aerobics class may be the best way to get a full-body workout, and you don't even need to know how to swim. Like any aerobics class, upbeat music and being with a group of people can make exercising more enjoyable and keep you motivated! Before choosing a class, make sure it is appropriate to your level of fitness and ability. Go and watch a class before you attend.

your swimming programme

To improve your aerobic fitness steadily, aim to swim two to three times a week.

weeks 1–2

Start by swimming twice in the first two weeks, say on Monday and Friday or Tuesday and Thursday, so that you have a day or two to rest in between. Aim to stay in the pool for about 30 minutes. Swim one length of the pool at your own pace, then rest for one minute or until your breath returns. Swim 10 lengths.

weeks 3–4

You have already started to make swimming part of your weekly routine. Make sure you still swim twice a week, and now think about adding an extra 5 lengths to each swim. Still rest for up to one minute after each length. You will be surprised how quickly you can swim this new distance. You may be in the pool more than 30 minutes when you first increase your lengths, but I guarantee that by the end of week 4 you will be swimming 15 lengths in 30 minutes. If, as you get fitter, you feel up to swimming 2 lengths before you need to rest, give it a try. If you are swimming with a friend, see who can finish first. The last to finish brings the healthy after-swim snack next session!

weeks 5–6

Increase your swimming to 2 lengths at a time, if you haven't done so already, before resting for one minute. In week 6, swim 4 lengths before taking your minute's rest. You will still swim 15 lengths, but now you are pushing your fitness and increasing the number of lengths you swim in each set. If you are swimming with a friend you can chat as you swim, and spend quality time while getting fit.

weeks 7–8

Now introduce more lengths and increase the number of lengths in your swim sets before you take that well-earned minute's rest. Swim 5 lengths now before you rest, and aim to swim 20 lengths in total. Try swimming a different stroke for each length, to stop you getting bored and also use different muscles. See how much further you can swim without needing a rest once you increase your fitness.

weeks 9–10

You should now be noticing changes in your fitness and your waistline! Introducing a float can vary your lengths and make you train your arms and legs harder. Most pools will have floats available – just ask the lifeguard. This is also a great way to improve your cardiovascular fitness. Hold onto a float with both hands and propel yourself through the water by only kicking your legs. Aim for 5 lengths before you take your minute's rest. It may sound like an easy option, but if you give it a go your legs won't agree, as they are doing all the work without help from your arms! For the next 5 lengths swim again, then repeat the 2 sets.

weeks 11–12

Another way to use your float is to hold it between your knees and swim using just your arms to pull you through the water. Swim your regular set of 5 lengths, alternating with 5 lengths with the float between your knees. Take rests as you need them – you will soon be increasing the number of lengths you can swim with just your arms as you get stronger. To have a mixed workout over the week, vary your programme each day. One day just swim, one day swim with the float in your hands, and one day alternate all three options – a length swimming, a length swimming with legs only and a length with arms only.

when to go
Choose a time of day which suits you but make sure you have eaten. Don't exercise for at least two hours after eating, as this will make you feel nauseous. Make sure you sip water during exercise but don't drink too much – it is more important to drink regularly throughout the day to avoid dehydration rather than too much all in one go.

getting back to fitness: taking it outdoors
Walking is no soft option. You can actually burn more calories walking than running, if you vary your walking speed and style. When you are suffering from back pain, walking gets you moving without the impact and jarring that is associated with running, while still getting you out in the fresh air. It's also free!

When you are in pain and maybe off work and practising active rest (see page 49), you can take a short walk a few times a day to make sure you keep moving. It may only be out into the garden at first, but then aim to walk further, perhaps to the local shop to buy a newspaper. Try using a pedometer – which counts the number of steps you take – and see if you can increase the number of steps you take each day.

'I thought back pain was part of old age but I was happy to be proved wrong. Swimming and walking have become part of my retirement routine and I even got a dog to make sure I have to walk at least twice a day.'

Sam, Yorkshire

fitting in exercise

- Get up 30 minutes earlier in the morning and walk to the station or the next bus stop along.
- Get off the bus two stops early and walk the rest of the way. If you can, walk to work.
- If you are not a morning person, take a walk after your evening meal rather than slumping in front of the TV. You can always record your favourite programme to watch when you get back.
- Take a walk before dinner or breakfast and work up an appetite. If you are out before breakfast at the weekend, bring home a treat of fresh croissants or bread.

The simple routine below will build up visible pace and stamina in only a few weeks. Alternatively, you may prefer to start on a treadmill or cross-trainer at the gym. Both of these prepare your body for exercise with less impact, and also mean that you will not be stranded should you feel the need to stop. This allows the body to adapt gradually to the stresses of exercise and helps you to avoid injury and making your back pain worse.

When walking, try to maintain a good posture from head to toe, with your head up and shoulders back, keeping your steps steady so you can keep up an even pace. Swinging your arms helps speed up your pace, and to progress as you get fitter you can swing your arms while holding weights. Make sure you have supportive footwear or trainers. Any running shop can give you advice on the right trainer for your foot type, which considers the shape and width of your foot and the height of your arch.

After you've tried the walking programme, you could progress to a mixed speed programme, where you mix periods of brisk walking with periods of slow walking, gradually increasing the duration of the brisk walk and decreasing the frequency of the slow walk.

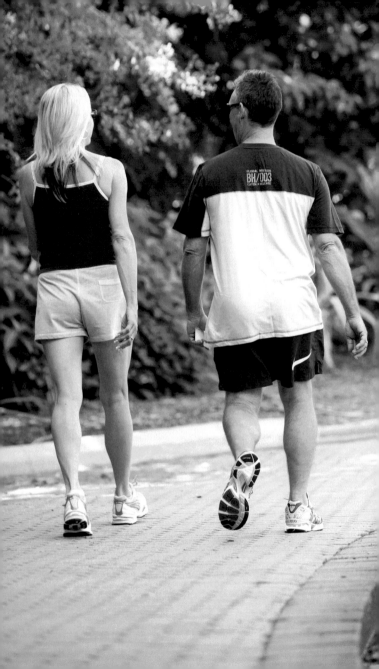

walk safe

It is important that you plan to walk on routes that are safe. This includes walking when it is light and in places which are busy and not secluded if you plan to walk on your own. Leave a note at home with the time you left for your walk, where you are going and when you are due home. Take your mobile phone with you so you are always in contact.

walking programme

weeks 1–2

Start by walking every day. This may be as simple as walking to the station, getting off the bus one stop early or walking to buy your lunch. Taking the stairs instead of the lift also counts as walking and may be possible more than once a day.

weeks 3–4

You have already added walking into your routine without taking up any extra time in weeks 1 and 2. Now think about adding an extra 15 minute walk into each day. This may be part of your route to work, to the shops or to a friend's home for coffee. You could offer to walk a neighbour's dog or give a new mother a break by taking her baby for a walk.

weeks 5–6

Increase your daily walking time to 20 minutes in week 5 and 30 minutes in week 6. You can use this time to switch off and have time to yourself, or if you prefer make phone calls and catch up with all those friends you never get round to calling back. Better still, get a friend to walk with you and spend quality time while walking.

weeks 7–8

Now you have an established routine of daily walking, it is time to speed things up a little. Introduce swinging your arms and focus on striding out as you walk. See how much further you can walk once you increase your pace. A pedometer will help you monitor your distance. Alternatively you could simply use a route you have walked previously in 30 minutes and aim to walk beyond the original finish point.

weeks 9–10

You should now be noticing changes in your fitness and waistline. You are ready to progress, and introducing uphill and downhill walking is a great way to improve your cardiovascular fitness. Find a hill either in a park or on a street, and walk up without stopping. Use the walk back down to get your breath back. You will still be working your muscles, just in a different way. You can make this a 15 minute part of your work-out – walking to and from the hill is a good warm-up and cool-down.

weeks 11–12

Another way to progress is to walk while holding weights. These don't have to cost money and can be two tins of beans! Walk your regular routes and focus on your pace and arm swing. To make sure your grip remains strong, secure the weights to your hands with loops of elastic: slip the loop over your hand and place the can of beans under the elastic in your palm. To have a mixed workout over the week, vary your programme each day – one day with weights, one day with hills and one day on the flat.

running/jogging programme

Starting to run is just as easy to achieve as the walking programme – it just depends on what you set yourself as a goal. Back pain doesn't stop you running unless it is severe, and if you monitor your back pain as you get fitter you will be able to run as much as you like. All the advice already given about starting any form of exercise is just as important before starting to run, and it is particularly important to get the right trainers. Any good running shop can give you advice on the right trainer for you.

Aim to follow this programme three times a week to see the best results in your fitness.

week 1

Walk for 5 minutes, swinging your arms and keeping up a quick, steady pace. Then jog at an easy pace for one minute. Repeat this 4 times and to finish add an extra 5 minute walk to cool down. If you can, persuade a friend to train with you, or failing that get them to be your coach and to time your walks and runs. They will soon be running with you when they see your fitness improving.

week 2

Walk for 4 minutes, then jog for 2 minutes. Repeat this 4 times, adding your cool-down walk at the end for 5 minutes. If you have a dog or can borrow one from a neighbour, they will love the run/walk and keep you company into the bargain.

week 3

This is the week your runs become longer than your walks! Start by walking for 3 minutes, then jog for 4 minutes. Repeat this 4 times. Now your timing buddy will really wish they had started running when you did, and your neighbour's dog will want a rest!

week 4

Not much walking this week! Start with a 2 minute walk, then jog for 6 minutes. Repeat this 4 times. Now you are jogging for 20 minutes altogether: who would have thought that 4 weeks ago?

week 5

Walk for 2 minutes to warm up and then increase your jogging time to 8 minutes. Repeat 3 times. Now you are jogging for longer, it's time to focus on your posture. Relax your shoulders, and keep your breathing steady. Try breathing in through your nose and out through your mouth. This will help warm the air before it gets to your lungs and stop your chest from feeling tight.

weeks 6–7

Now it's time to speed things up a little. Introduce swinging your arms and focus on striding out as you jog. See how quickly your jog can become a run once you increase your pace. Many mobile phones now have built-in GPS which will help you monitor your distance, or simply use a route you have jogged previously and aim to run beyond the original finish point. Start by walking for 2 minutes and then jog/run for 10 minutes. Repeat 3 times.

week 8

Congratulations for sticking at your running programme and making it to week 8. From now on, walk for 5 minutes at the start and finish of your run to warm up and cool down. Try to jog/run for 20 minutes between your walks for your first 2 sessions this week and 30 minutes at the end of the week.

Now you have become a runner, aim to run for 30 minutes 3 times a week. Your fitness and stamina will continue to improve. If you set your goal as running a race for charity, book your place now, as you are well on the way to achieving your first 5 kilometres!

exercises for your back

These are specific exercises for your back that will strengthen your body and help you to manage and reduce your back pain. You may have done some of them before and others may be new to you. When you are in pain you may be nervous about exercising, but remember, if you take it slowly you will not harm yourself or make your pain worse. It is important to pace yourself (see page 46) and be guided by your body as to how many repetitions of each exercise are right for you. You will be able to do more as you get stronger and as your back pain gets better.

choosing your exercises

Here are some suggestions for different stages of your back pain.

When you are in severe pain:

- consider the first week of the swimming or walking pro-grammes – both will help keep you moving but are gentle, and if you pace yourself will not make your pain worse

- pole dancing, especially lying down (page 104)
- transverse abdominis (page 96)
- the clam (page 93)
- pelvic floor (page 98)
- the cat stretch (page 105).

At this stage, do whatever you feel able to which does not increase the level of pain.

As things start to improve:

- pace yourself through the walking or swimming programmes as you feel able – though stay with week 1 for a week or two if that suits you
- the bug (page 100)
- leg press on gym ball (page 91)
- any two of the general exercises (pages 88–91).

Aim to exercise for 15 minutes every day if you feel able to.

As you are ready to progress:

- get moving with either the walking or swimming programme – alternate different weeks if you like variety – or start on the running programme
- the bug with arm floats and leg floats, or both if you can (pages 101–102)
- the plank (page 102)
- the hamstring curl (page 94)
- the bridge (page 95)
- the neural glide (page 112).

At this stage you can try any of the other exercises in this book, and aim to exercise for 15–30 minutes daily. You can do different exercises every day if you like, but by now you will probably have your favourites!

general exercises

press-ups

Press-ups are a great exercise to strengthen the muscles around your shoulders and upper back. You can adjust this exercise to your own level of fitness by using a wall to start with to make it easier, and then progress to a worktop or bench and finally to the floor as your back gets stronger.

1 Place your hands on a wall at chest height and spread them slightly wider than shoulder distance apart.

2 Slowly bend your elbows to move your chest towards the wall, then straighten your arms to push yourself away from the wall, making sure you don't arch your back.

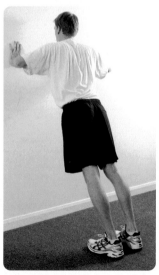

Easy against a wall

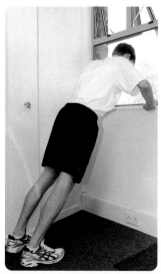

Harder against a window ledge or worktop

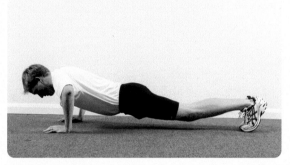

Difficult on the floor

squats

If you have back pain, your lifting technique is probably not as good as it could be (see page 41). Squats are a great way to strengthen your legs to help you lift properly. If your back is sore or you are unfit, start by gently standing and carefully sitting back down in a chair. You can progress as you become stronger. It is important to squat properly to make sure you don't hurt your knees. It also makes sure you work all the muscles in your legs and bottom without straining your back.

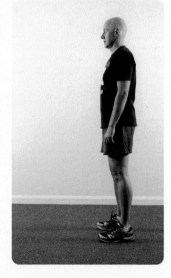

1 Stand with your feet hip distance apart and your weight equally placed on the balls of your feet and heels. Reach your arms out in front of you to help you balance.

2 Bend your knees and stick your bottom out behind you as if you are going to sit on a chair.

3 Make sure your knees and ankles are at 90 degrees, keeping your knees behind your toes. This makes sure you don't put too much weight onto the back of the kneecap.

4 Only squat as low as you can with good posture.

Repeat 5–10 times for 3 sets. Rest as you need to between sets.

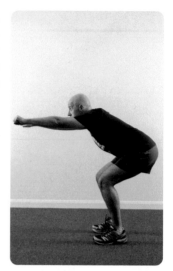

step-ups

You only need the bottom step for this exercise at home.

1 Use the banister or the wall for balance if you need to.

2 Step up with your right leg, ensuring your heel is on the step, then bring your left leg up alongside it.

3 Step down with your right leg, bringing the left foot to join it.

4 Repeat, leading with your left leg.

Repeat each leg 10 times for 3 sets.

If you can't step up because of back, leg or buttock pain, march on the spot, lifting your foot to the height of the step or lower if you need to. You will soon be able to step up.

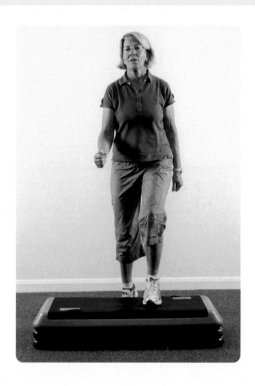

buttocks and legs

leg press on gym ball

what is a gym ball?
This is a large inflatable ball that you can use to help you stretch and exercise, and it also makes a great chair to encourage good posture. The taller you are, the bigger ball you will need. You can buy them from Argos, most large department stores and online. Expect to pay about £25 at most.

This exercise will help strengthen your legs and is really useful if you are weak or in pain. It is also a great way to start working on your single leg balance if you have had leg pain associated with nerve irritation or compression in your back.

1   Lie on your back with your hips and knees at 90 degrees, with your feet holding a gym ball off the floor and against a wall.

2   Keeping your back flat on the floor, push your feet into the ball to add some resistance, and roll it up and down the wall by slowly bending and straightening your knees.

3   Straighten your knees as far as you comfortably can – if you have sciatica don't try to straighten your knee fully. Be guided by your pain.

Repeat 10 times for 3 sets, first with both feet on the ball and then with each leg alone.

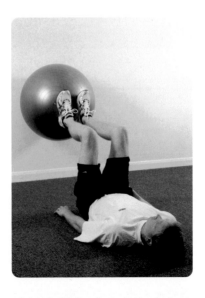

the clam

This is a great exercise to strengthen your glutes (buttock muscles), which are part of your outer core that supports the spine. The glutes help to control the position of the hip and can make exercising much easier when they are stronger.

1 Lie on your side with your arm underneath you outstretched in line with your trunk.

2 Rest your head on this arm.

3 Bend your hips and knees up to about 90 degrees and rest your top hand on the floor.

4 Draw your top hip downwards away from the top shoulder to create a small space between your waist and the floor or mat.

5 Breathe out and lift your top knee upwards, keeping your feet together.

6 Breathe in and lower your top knee onto your bottom leg.

Repeat 10 times as one set. As you get stronger you can add extra sets.

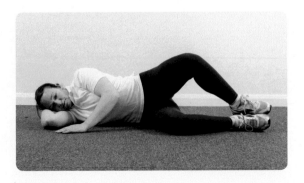

the hamstring curl

This is a great exercise to strengthen the back of your legs, your glutes (in your bottom) and your core muscles.

1 Lie on your back with your feet on a gym ball.

2 Keep your arms out to the sides to help you to balance.

3 Lift your bottom off the floor and balance your weight on your shoulder blades.

4 Bend your knees, bringing your heels to your bottom.

5 Straighten your knees again to the starting position.

6 If you get pain in your back, stop and start again with your pelvis in a lower position.

Repeat 10 times as one set, and aim for 3 sets.

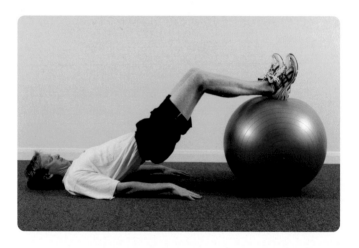

Variations:

- An easier option is to hold your position without bending your knees backwards and forwards. Squeeze the muscles in your bottom to keep you stable, but keep your knees soft.
- To make the exercise harder, move your hands closer to your body and then onto your chest. Keep the leg position the same.

the bridge

1 Lie flat on your back with your knees bent, your arms by your sides and feet flat on the floor.

2 Lift your bottom slowly off the floor, then lift your pelvis and slowly peel away your spine, level by level.

3 Squeeze your glutes gently and hold for 10 seconds.

4 Slowly lower your spine back to the floor, placing your pelvis down last.

Do 2 sets of 10 repetitions.

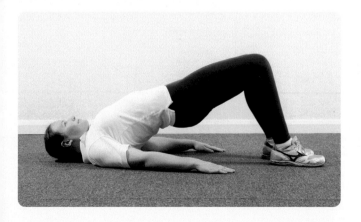

Variations:
- Use a cushion or ball to squeeze between your knees to work your inner thighs.
- To make this harder, once you have reached the top of the lift, lift one foot slowly off the floor and extend one knee, stretching your toes away from your body. Don't allow your pelvis to rock and keep the cushion or ball in place if using one. Hold for 2–5 seconds and then slowly lower the foot back to the floor. Repeat on the opposite leg, alternating until you have raised each leg 5 times.

trunk and low back (core stability exercises)

The muscles of the trunk and low back will usually have been weakened by back pain. In part 1 we looked at the muscular slings and deep core stability muscles that support your spine. The following exercises are the ones that your muscles need to create the strength and control to make a difference to your back pain.

transverse abdominis

This may be a slow and dull exercise, but it is one of the most important exercises you can learn if you have had back pain. It is the staple exercise of Pilates classes, and dancers have used it for years to maintain their core strength.

1 Lie on your back with your knees bent, your feet on the floor and your head supported on a small pillow or folded towel.

2 Relax the weight of your head into the pillow and lengthen the back of your neck by reaching the top of your head towards the wall behind you.

3 Gently draw your shoulder blades down towards your waist to relax your neck and shoulders.

4 Place your feet and knees hip distance apart and place your fingers on your lower tummy muscle.

5 Imagine your pelvis is a bucket of water. Tip it backwards to spill some water out of the back of the bucket and you will feel your back gently flatten onto the floor.

6 Now tip it forwards to spill some water out of the front of the bucket and you will feel your lower back arch slightly.

7 Find your 'neutral spine' position by resting the bucket halfway between these two movements.

8 Maintaining this neutral spine position, take a breath in, then slowly breathe out until you have no breath left.

9 At the end of your out breath you will feel your deep abdominal muscles engage under your fingers.

10 Maintain this muscle activation gently as you keep breathing in and out for up to ten breaths.

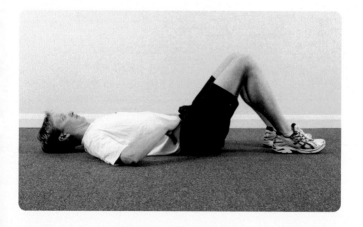

pelvic floor activation

the pelvic floor

The pelvic floor is an important part of your core stability muscles. It's a dynamic platform, similar to a trampoline, and its chief function is to support the pelvic and abdominal organs. It also controls continence. Obviously these are important functions, but you can also reduce back pain by training these muscles. A strengthened pelvic floor creates a more stable spine and supports your core muscles when you are lifting. This is better than holding your breath, which is what many of us do when we lift.

Pelvic floor exercises can be difficult to get right as the muscles are not directly visible, but everyone with back pain, male and female, should do them. A fully functioning pelvic floor is not appreciated until you lose it! You can exercise these muscles in a variety of situations: on the bus, queuing, on the phone, or waiting for the kettle to boil. Performing pelvic floor exercises in different positions will change how they feel, so try to find a position that you find easier and which gives you the greatest sensation or better quality of contraction. It is also important to make sure you are not holding your breath, bearing down, or squeezing your buttocks or tummy muscles too much.

If you are struggling with locating or exercising your pelvic floor, ask for a referral to a physiotherapist – all physiotherapists routinely teach pelvic floor exercises to people with back pain. For helpful products visit www.mobilishealthcare.com or www.neenpelvichealth.com. You might also like to look at www.bladderandbowelfoundation.org where you will get more advice on finding your pelvic floor.

For women:

1   Remember, whilst this is the muscle that stops your urine flow, you must not practise trying to do so.

2   Think about squeezing on a tampon, or lifting yourself away from your underwear.

3   You can insert a finger into your vagina and squeeze as an alternative way to feel your pelvic floor.

4   Pelvic floor trainers are available and easy to use if you are finding this exercise difficult. However, you must be using your muscles properly or they won't work. They are sold with the maternity products.

For men:

1   Imagine you are walking into a cold river and you don't want to get your testicles wet.

2   Gently using your pelvic floor muscle, lift your testicles up and away from your underwear.

3   Remember, whilst this is the muscle that stops your urine flow, you must not practise trying to do so. However, you do use it at the end of urination.

Duration and repetitions:
To train the pelvic floor for both strength and endurance functions two methods are recommended:

- Try long, strong contractions one after the other with about ten seconds' rest in between. Hold each for as long as possible and see how many you can perform before tiring.

- You should also practise short, sharp and quick contractions, again until you get tired.

It is important that you do both types of exercise otherwise your muscle control and strength will not improve. How well you perform the exercises will vary – the time of day and being pre-menstrual if you're female will have an effect. In just a few weeks you will see improvements in the quality, duration and number of contractions.

the bug

This is a progression from the transverse abdominis exercise described above, and will help you strengthen your deep core stability muscles gently but effectively.

1 Lie on your back with your arms reaching up towards the ceiling and your hips and knees bent to 90 degrees. If this feels too difficult, you can support your legs on a gym ball or on the arm of a sofa. You will still benefit your core without straining your back, and can progress as you feel able.

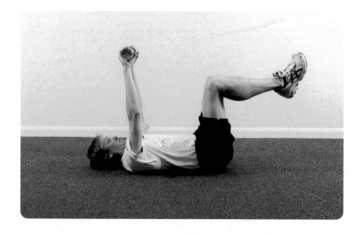

2 Make sure your spine is flattened gently against the floor and your pelvic floor is lifted.

3 Hold this position as you gently breathe in and out.

4 You should feel this in your tummy but not in your back. If you have back pain, wait until you are stronger or reduce the time you hold the position.

Repeat 3 times for 10 breaths, resting between each set.

Variations:
- **Arm floats:** as you breathe out, slowly raise your left arm over your head, then breathe in and return your arm to the start position. Alternate each arm for 30 seconds, increasing to one minute as you become stronger.

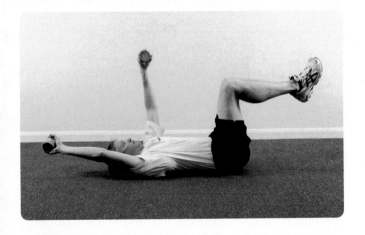

- **Leg floats:** as you breathe out, slowly lower your left foot towards the floor, but only as far as you can while keeping a neutral spine. Breathe in and return the hip to the start position. Alternate legs for 30 seconds, increasing to one minute as you become stronger.

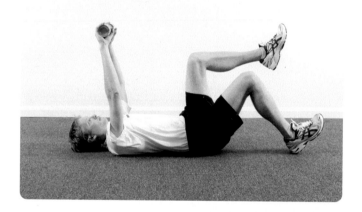

the plank

The plank will strengthen your tummy without making it bigger. You should never feel pain in your back with this exercise. If you do, don't progress on to the variations until your strength improves.

1 Lie on your tummy with your forearms flat on the floor in front of you and your elbows directly under your shoulders.

2 Push yourself up onto your forearms, moving your tummy away from the floor and your tailbone towards your feet. Keep your knees on the floor so you are balanced with a flat back and parallel to the floor. Using a mirror will help you monitor your position.

3 Hold this position for one minute, then lower yourself down.

Repeat 3 times.

Make sure you keep your upper arms at 90 degrees to your body and your shoulders directly over your elbows. Squeezing your bottom also helps to keep your balance and stops your back aching.

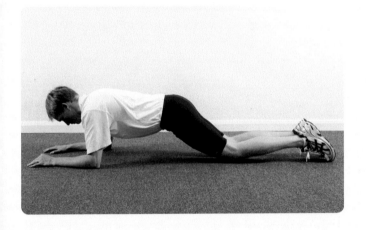

Variations: The best variation to this exercise is also a progression. Again, you should not feel any pain in the lower back.

- Once you have pushed yourself up, reach forward with each hand, alternating for 10 reps. This makes the exercise less stable and means you have to work your muscles much harder.
- Alternatively, alternate extending your knees while squeezing your glutes for 10 reps.

spinal flexibility

pole dancing

These pelvic tilts are great for keeping your back and pelvis loose and are a good place to start when you have a flare-up.

1 Stand with your hands on your hips and your feet hip distance apart, keeping your knees soft and slightly bent.

2 Imagine your pelvis is a bucket filled with water.

3 Ensure that you keep your spine straight and that all the movement comes from your pelvis and the bottom of your spine.

4 Then try any or all of the following:

- **Pelvic tilts:** tilt your pelvis forwards and backwards as if you are tipping water out of the front and the back of the bucket.
- **Side tilts:** tilt your pelvis side to side as if you are tipping water out of the left and right sides of the bucket.
- **Pelvic circles:** combining the pelvic and side tilts, put your hands on your hips and circle your pelvis as if you are swilling water around the top of the bucket but not letting any spill out.

Variations: These exercises are versatile for all abilities and levels of pain:

- You can do them all in many positions – sitting on a gym ball, standing, kneeling on all fours, and lying down. Use whichever position is most comfortable for you, but aim to be able to do the exercise both sitting down and standing up.

- If your back is stiff or sore, this is a great one to try lying down before you get up in the morning.

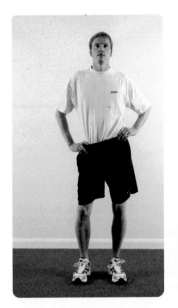 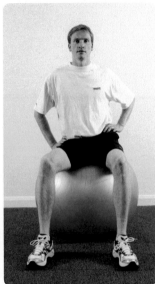

the cat stretch

This is a gentle exercise you can do even when you are in severe pain. It will help restore movement to your spine and release muscle spasm.

1 Kneel on all fours with your knees hip distance apart, and your hands shoulder width apart.

2 Imagine your pelvis is a bucket filled with water.

3 Tilt your pelvis forwards and backwards as if you are tipping water out of the front and back of the bucket.

4 Ensure you allow your mid spine to curl and uncurl as you move your pelvis.

There is no limit to how many times you can do this exercise – it is gentle and can be repeated little and often.

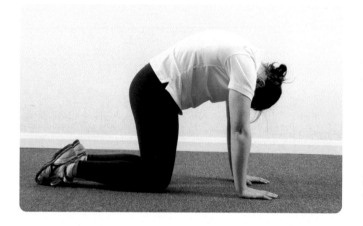

crucifix stretch

This is a great stretch for the lumbar spine and hips, while also stretching the buttocks, back muscles and hamstrings.

1 Lie on your back with your arms stretched out at right angles and your legs straight, as if you were on a crucifix. Keep both arms in contact with the floor at all times.

2 Lift your right leg 5 cm off the floor and swing your leg over and across your left leg so the toes on your right foot are sliding towards your left hand. Only swing your leg as far as you can comfortably go. As your pain reduces and your flexibility increases you will get more rotation in your spine.

3 Return your right leg to the start position and repeat with the left leg.

Do 2 sets of 10–15 repetitions.

Variations: If your flexibility is poor or if you have had a flare-up of low back pain, bend your knees, keeping your feet on the floor, and roll your knees from side to side.

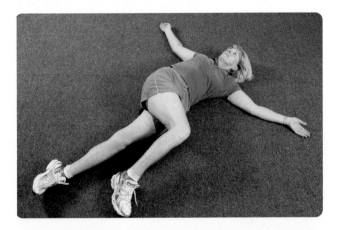

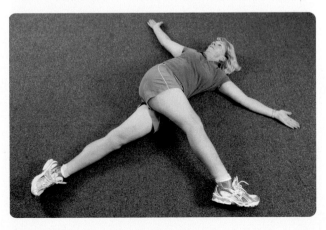

upper back and neck stretches

These simple exercises will help to stretch the muscles around your neck gently and allow you to maintain a full range of movement and good posture.

hold–relax stretch

1 Gently push the side of your head into your hand and hold for 10 seconds.

2 Stop pushing into your hand and gently stretch your neck, moving your ear towards your shoulder. You can use your hand to increase the stretch if it feels comfortable to do so. Hold this stretch for 5 seconds and repeat on the other side.

3 You can do this as many times as you need to make your neck feel loose.

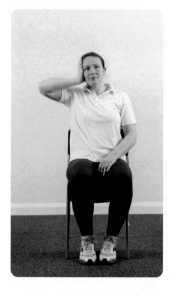 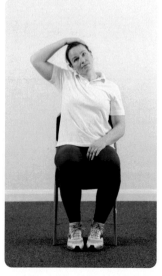

Variation: This same stretch can be used to help rotation in your neck:

1 Gently push your cheek into your hand as you try to turn your head.

2 Hold for 10 seconds, relax and then turn your head further to the right or left.

3 Repeat this hold and relax process until you feel you have reached your comfortable limit of movement.

chin tucks

This is a great exercise to improve your posture and reduce stiffness at the base of your neck and the top of your spine. You can do this sitting at work or lying in bed.

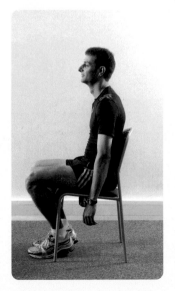
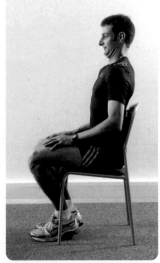

1 Make sure you have a good sitting or lying posture.

2 Drop your chin slightly to give yourself a double chin and keep your head in this position.

3 Gently push the tip of your tongue into the roof of your mouth.

4 If you are sitting, move your head backwards; if lying down, push your head into the supporting surface.

5 Hold this position for 2–3 seconds then relax your tongue and double chin.

6 Never push into pain and keep it slow and gentle at all times.

Variation: Make this harder by working with resistance:

1 Lie on your back with your head on a firm pillow or a gym ball.

2 Push the back of your head into the pillow or the ball and relax.

3 Slowly turn your head from side to side as you maintain your double chin.

end of the day stretch

Lying on a rolled towel for 15–20 minutes every night before you go to sleep is a great stretch both for your spine between the shoulder blades and for your chest muscles. If this area is stiff or tight it will affect the movement in your shoulders.

1 Roll up a towel so it has a diameter of 10–15 cm and secure it with rubber bands.

2 Lie on a bed with the towel lengthways down your spine, from the base of your neck to the middle of your back.

3 Raise your arms to either side of your head and let them rest on the bed. If this is too much of a stretch, rest your arms on pillows to reduce the pull across your chest.

Variation: You can achieve the same stretch by lying over a gym ball.

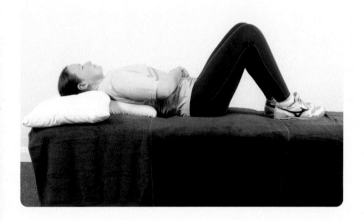

nerve sliding and gliding

These are important exercises if you have or have had sciatica (see page 15). Pacing is especially important when you do these exercises, as too many will make your leg pain worse. The aim is to encourage the nerve to move and slide normally again. This movement is often restricted by muscle spasm and pain and at worst by a disc bulge. The exercises encourage better circulation in the nerve and more normal movement in the body as the protective spasm in your muscle is reduced.

Do one of these exercises but not both. Try them on different days and see which works best for you and your sciatica.

gliding in lying

1 Lie curled up on your pain-free side with your head supported on a pillow.

2 Slowly and gently nod your head, taking your chin to your chest.

3 You should not feel any pain, but feeling a stretch in the spine is fine.

4 Progress by keeping your head still and slowly bending and straightening your top leg. Move as far as you can without pain.

Repeat no more than 20 times. Do fewer reps and keep to a smaller range if your leg pain is severe.

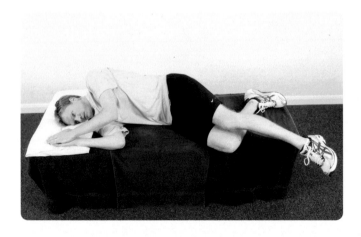

gliding in standing

1 Stand with the foot of your painful leg on a chair.

2 Slowly lean forwards, sliding your hands down the outside of your calf.

3 Only move in a pain-free range and repeat no more than 20 times.

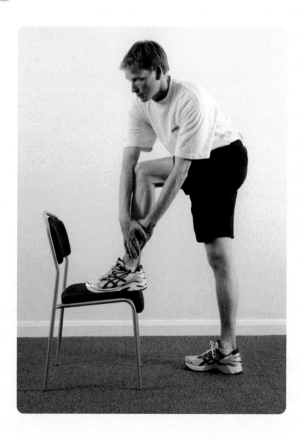

balance exercises

These are great exercises to strengthen your ankles and improve your balance. It is important to do these if you have had leg pain and weakness due to a nerve being compressed in your back.

balancing on a wobble cushion

You can buy wobble cushions from exercise equipment shops or online from www.physiosupplies.co.uk. For this exercise you can even use an inflatable mattress to create an unstable surface to balance on.

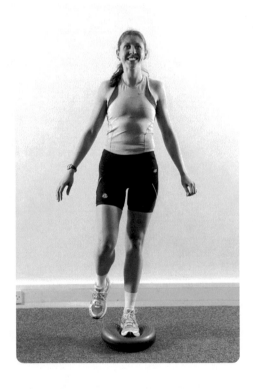

1 Stand with both feet on the wobble cushion, keeping your knees soft. Allow yourself to wobble a little, as the point of the exercise is to control the wobble without falling off the cushion.

2 You may need to place the cushion near a wall or kitchen worktop to help you balance – when you get stronger you can try to balance without support.

3 To make it harder, stand on one leg.

You can practise standing on one leg every time you clean your teeth – a great way to make it a daily exercise with very little effort.

ankle flicks

All you need for this is a tennis ball and a wall. This exercise is important if you have had sciatica, as the nerve that supplies the muscle around the ankle may have been affected.

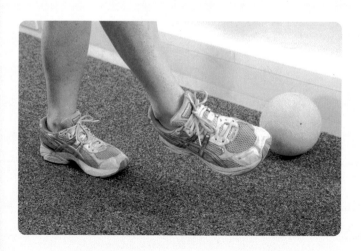

1 Stand on one leg next to a wall.

2 Using a tennis ball, kick the ball with the side of your foot against the wall.

3 You can work the muscles on the inside and the outside of your ankle by a simple change of position and kicking with the inner or outer part of the foot.

4 You can do a similar exercise using a resistance band, so you can still do the exercise if your back pain means you need to sit down.

find out more

back pain

BackCare – the Charity for Healthier Backs
www.backcare.org.uk
Helpline: 0845 130 2704

Back in Action
www.backinaction.co.uk

Balance Performance Physiotherapy
www.balancephysio.com

Chartered Society of Physiotherapy
www.csp.org.uk

Health and Safety Executive – Back Pain in the Workplace
www.hse.gov.uk/msd/backpain

Health and Safety Executive – Better Backs Campaign
www.hse.gov.uk/betterbacks

RealHealth Institute
www.realhealth.org.uk

CBT
British Association for Cognitive and Behavioural Therapists
http://www.babcp.com

Mood Gym
http://moodgym.anu.edu.au

Living Life to the Full
www.livinglifetothefull.com